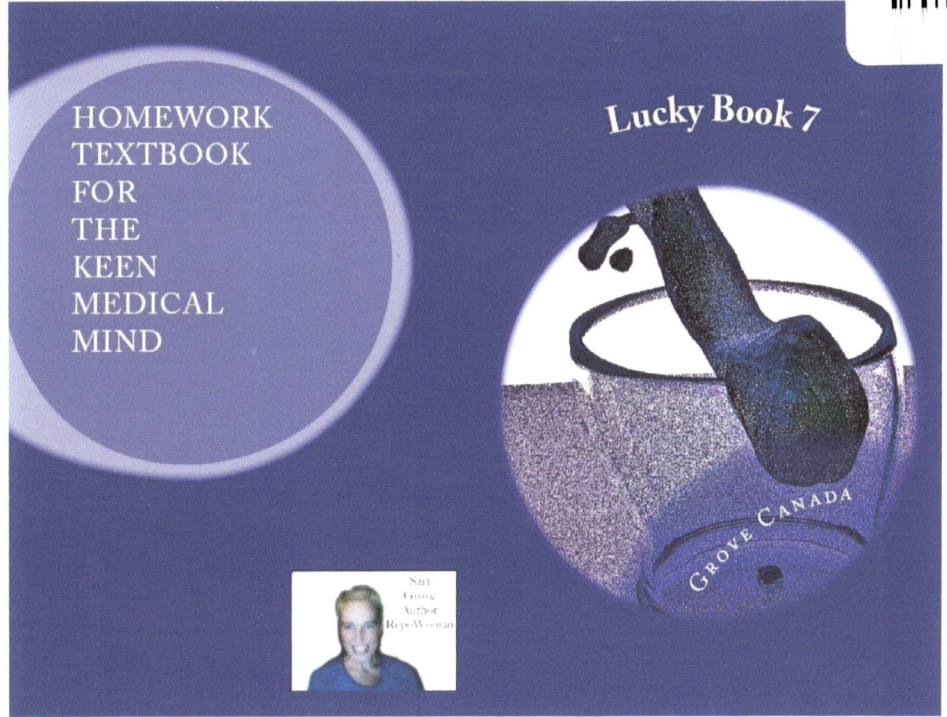

HOMEWORK
TEXTBOOK
FOR
THE
KEEN
MEDICAL
MIND

Lucky Book 7

GROVE CANADA

Table of Contents:

Rules, Protocols, Lessons Learned, Cemented Ideas...   8

DIY Mammo: 9

How to get the Iodine you need to shrink your breast lump...   20

I'm an artist who innovates in the Medical Arts...   28

RepoWoman is a nonsurgical breast cancer lump removal
protocol...   31

Joseph Grove   38

Hints on how to figure out what is in the drugs you are taking, &
where they fit in on the Grove Body Part Chart, which will help you
to know what they do to your body, so you can antidote them or
prevent getting addicted to the drug...   39

The flow of elements...   43

Salt...   43

Water...   47

So we are stuck on flow...   51

Chicken or Egg   53

Very short religious bio...   56

In the Brain...   56

Mustard Gas   60

The chemicals used in older fashioned photographic processing
can have a tendency to produce Lung Cancer...For example,
Aluminum Chloride, a hardener(at the end of the fixing process for
printing), has an affinity to clog up the Lungs & Lymph node
system...   62

(from my blog)(a R.I.P. article)   62

SOMEONE TOLD ME ABOUT GICLEES & I THOUGHT IT WAS A
SURE THING!(WARNING:SAD ARTICLE)   62

Picture shows a tree's root system on a little hilly area,   80

Cycling...Hitting your head with hemet on...Concussion...After
effects...Let's look at one possibility angle of impact & how it
could affect the human...   81

(Detour   81

Cycling, coma and living with a brain injury   81

by Nick Mercer),   81

Oh I forgot to add...Generally in most concussion, there is a rise in
Potassium levels, with a commensurate drop of Aurum...   83

If the fall is to the back of the head, on the right side, the Selenium side, of the Occipital lobe(& that area fails), then you get Sulphur Sugar dominance in the Pancreas & eyes & of course that section of the Occipital Lobe...   85

Revisiting the order of things...   86

So if tea & milk are happy together, & they marry easily, or just date well, then we are maybe confirming the thought that MINUS elements come BEFORE plus elements on the Chart, & in the FLOW of the Body Parts...   87

Remembrance Day, Veteran's Day, Armistice Day, Day of the Dead...   87

The technical term is called RHABDOMYOLYSIS...(the link above takes you to a Mayo clinic explanation of that)...Leg cramps...You can also duplicate this burning of muscle effect, the leg cramp thing, by exercising too much without eating enough...So, theoretically, the cure for leg cramps would be to put some cholesterol back in your body, stop taking Crestor or whatever Statin you are taking(aspirin counts, as do asthma drugs), or stop exercising so much, or sit on a concrete rock or concrete chair to osmote the natural Aluminum there...   89

Back to the order of things for a moment...   90

About chemistry...   90

As a sidenote: There are now some metals that have a low burning threshold, so low that they are UNDER the 800 degree mark of a candle flame...   93

I noticed...   94

Alcohol is a heavy duty Hydrogen supplier...   95

"Canadian Park Ranger rescue:"Come over here, get into my truck!"...   95

End of this section Wed. Nov. 12, 2014 12:02 pm Eastern Standard Time...   95

The RepoWoman suggested schedule idea plan...   96

Explanation: Wake up whenever you wake up naturally, no alarm clock or time constraints or guilt...Whenever you feel rested enough to get out of bed, that is when you begin...   96

Walk means walk...   97

Reward...   99

Grocery Shop...   100

DIY Chemo Notes:Read Book 6   101

RepoWoman for the BASIC DIY chemo protocol...   101

An UPPER like Licorice Root combined with a DOWNER like Madagascar Periwinkle, can cause an up & down effect in your body...   102

Ok end of the RepoWoman advice...ish...for now...   103

Third Dimension...Of paired brain parts...(where are they & which one is which)???   104

Front of brain or back of brain...   106

Left side of brain or right side of brain...   106

Top of brain or bottom of brain...   106

(Because the brain criss-crosses to the body part because the criss-cross is stronger...   107

Families of elements that are similar but stronger or weaker than...   110

So now we know that stronger MINUS elements are HOTTER...112

We should also assume that stronger Plus elements are COLDER...So Lithium should be COLDER than Lead(Plomb Pb)...   113

Chrysanthemum tea...   114

Zig Zag: 115

Index credits...What follows is a flow (Feng Shui) of thoughts that are variably UNedited...This is HOW I come about getting new ideas & A-Ha moments...It is an artist's technique sometimes called Abstract Expressionism, (Les Automatistes) Automatism...   115

Variability of weights of things(density actually)   123

Grape on a Vine (it looks like a Chardonnay, mustard coloured)124

Some of Sari Grove's raw in process artworks pictures(the underneath that is no longer visible once the works are finished)...See more at http://www.grovecanada.ca   128

A second look at gender Polarity in brain & body parts...   132

the left side of the brain part   132

controls the right body part   132

the top of the brain part in a pair   132

controls the Bottom of the feet for example   132

the front brain part in a pair   132

controls the minus element ie the female back of the body   132

Frontal lobe r l means...   133

that the frontal lobe has 2 sides a right side &   133

a left side   133

are paired... Broca's sits to the front & Wernicke's area sits to the back (of the brain)   133 go left again go left again(you are now into a SPIN) Fibonacci Alan Turing...credits.   134

other things that need more pondering...   135

(Worms, like the Salmonella Typhi worm, can hole up in your breast lung tissue & cause Cancers-which is what makes cancer extra-tricky to solve-you have to deworm yourself-Hulled hemp seeds, like a teaspoon, are powerful dewormers-just remember they also cause memory loss, so be careful & use JUDICIOUSLY)...   136

I am a member of ArtConcrete group through Yahoo Groups...Here is an excerpt of a conversation about using Aragonite sand from pet stores for your marble dust in concrete recipes...(or just homemade marble recipes...See our website http://www.grovecanada.ca for some of those recipes we invented ourselves!)   137

Here is an email letter I wrote a while back while I was working on Book 3 of this series(Grove Health Science Series)...   139

"http://youtu.be/2IULrs6J9jU This is the video that explains the chart...   139

From September 2009, an early version of the chart...   145

Food for thought...My rough notes to myself(I email ideas to myself,in the middle of the night, from bed, from my iPhone Notes app, to my Fastmail account, so I can see them in big on my desktop computer in the morning...)   145

3 sections(are there really 3 parts- the brain, the body part, & then the limbs???)   146

(that the body flow goes BACKWARDS or UP the spinal column to the Brain-that the body sorts through good & bad stuff when eating, excretes what it doesn't want, then what remains gets to go up the spinal cord, upwards to the brain stem, which is why only the most select items make it up to the brain-like Cilantro for instance Does make it up to the brain...)   148 (that the new e-cigarettes do NOT burn paper, so NO ash Bismuth goes into the Lungs...Is it the ASH in regular cigarettes that causes buildup of gunk?)   148

(That ingesting Lead things like a potato or a carrot, builds that part of the body, like the Bones, & then that area will look bigger & be bigger...So like if you want to build your breastplate skeleton "look"...Eat things that are Plus elements in the Thyroid...)   149

Repeat what we know about Polarity...   149

Because brain stem direction flows UP the back of the spine into brain, brain parts are backwards to body parts in polarity or direction...   150

(idea:that releasing Phosphorus by masturbation lowers testosterone levels or estrogen levels, also thus lowering violent impulses, since violence has been linked to high testosterone levels...)   150

Go slow to go fast...   151

Slow down to go faster!(planning to drive slowly in heavy traffic or construction relieves the anger associated with that trip & makes the rest of the day seem to go faster & easier...Plus going slower in ALL things that you do enables fewer mistakes & edits later...Which is faster in the long run...)   151

(that the Bismuth in Pepto Bismol is great hangover remedy because much of the liquids we drink contain Fluorine which causes diarrhea & vomiting...Bismuth antidotes fluorine...)   151

(that when you "black out" when drinking heavily, it is the Hydrogen just putting you to sleep...Which is why insomniacs like drinking...water, alcohol, whatever that contains Hydrogens...Oxygens wake you up...)   152

(that people of African origin have great teeth due to high Ash Bismuth consumption because they eat foods more likely to be blackened over a flame...Consider eating more barbecued foods if your teeth are thin over-fluoridated looking?)   152

p.s.This book(& all the others too) gets edited & updated from time to time...Raw versions as we progress are available all the way along because that is the world we live in today...Immediacy is the norm & people don't want to wait 10 years anymore for medical information to be released...   152

Water flowing backwards...   153

Wonder when dentist's will stop overfluoridating our Lake Ontario water supply???   153

(Wed. Nov. 26, 2014)   155

The Making of a prosthetic left hand...Sari Grove   155

The world breaks everyone and afterward many are strong in the broken places. But those that will not break it kills. It kills the very good and the very gentle and the very brave impartially. If you are none of these you can be sure it will kill you too but there will be no special hurry.
Ernest Hemingway, A Farewell to Arms, 1929

Rules, Protocols, Lessons Learned, Cemented Ideas...

DIY Mammo:

Step by step DIY Mammogram at home...

So you have a lump in your breast...Sigh...Maybe it's been called Breast cancer...Maybe not...Either way you want to get rid of it...
Maybe you are following my RepoWoman protocol to get rid of it...

See RepoWoman:Book VI of the Grove Health Science series for our DIY Nonsurgical Breast Cancer (or Otherwise) Lump Removal Protocol...

Ok, so first, take your top off, go somewhere with good light(kitchen is good by the stove),
set your camera to MACRO with FLASH ON,

 hold your camera pretty close to where your lump is,
like 2 inches away, & take a picture...
Check it...You may need a few tries to get the whole area where your lump is in the picture...

Upload your pictures to your Mac computer to iPhoto...(Sorry, I only use a Mac...)
(but maybe the other computer editing programs will be sort of similar?)

In Edit Mode, in Quick Fixes, Click ENHANCE...

In EFFECTS, Click Boost as many times as you can, for me it goes 9 times total...

In Adjust, SLIDE the sliders for Definition, Shadows, Highlights, Sharpness-ALLTHE WAY TO THE RIGHT...

Still in ADJUST, Slide the CONTRAST & SATURATION sliders all the way to the right too...

FINALLY,in ADJUST, SLIDE THE BLUE_YELLOW SLIDER ALL THE WAY TO THE BLUEST...(in my case far left)

You will see your lump now under the skin...

You will see its shape & you will see its chemistry inside of it...

If the lump is relatively clear, then it is mostly just Calcium & Iron & it is benign...

If the lump has dark spots in it, like dark purple ants is how I see it, then you have Phosphorus & it is malignant...

Go read RepoWoman to see what to do next...

(Hint:One of the most important things you can do is start to take some form of very strong Licorice Root...

Licorice root is a highly absorbable COPPER that KILLS Phosphorus...

Killing Phosphorus means you kill spreadability...

The thing that makes cancer scary is spreadability, which is the Phosphorus stuff, which is like mold...

Taking the Licorice root(extract is strongest, tea is not bad, capsules are ok, boiling the herb is pretty good)handles the spread problem...

If you just control spread then all you will be left with is a lump...

A relatively benign lump...Not scary...

Read RepoWoman to get the rest of the protocol...

(If you buy a copy, that is neat for me, because even though the $1.99 Kindle price doesn't make me rich, it does feel good to see the tiny royalty reports...)

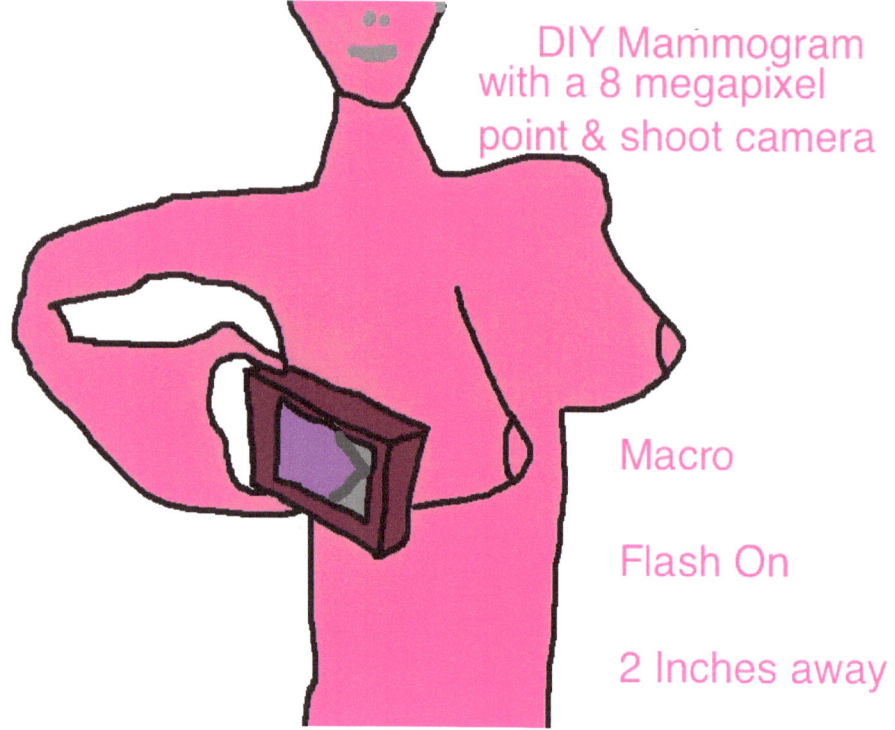

DIY Mammogram
with a 8 megapixel
point & shoot camera

Macro

Flash On

2 Inches away

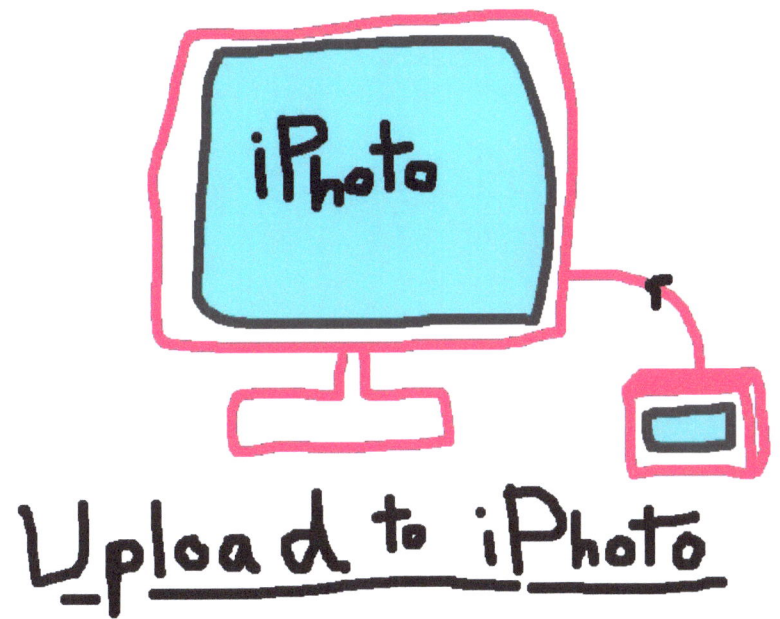

Upload to iPhoto

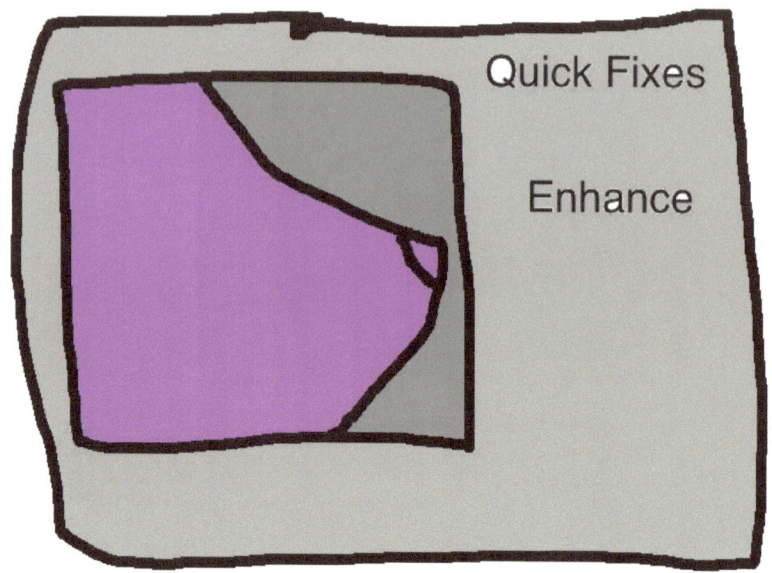

Quick Fixes

Enhance

In EDIT Mode: Enhance

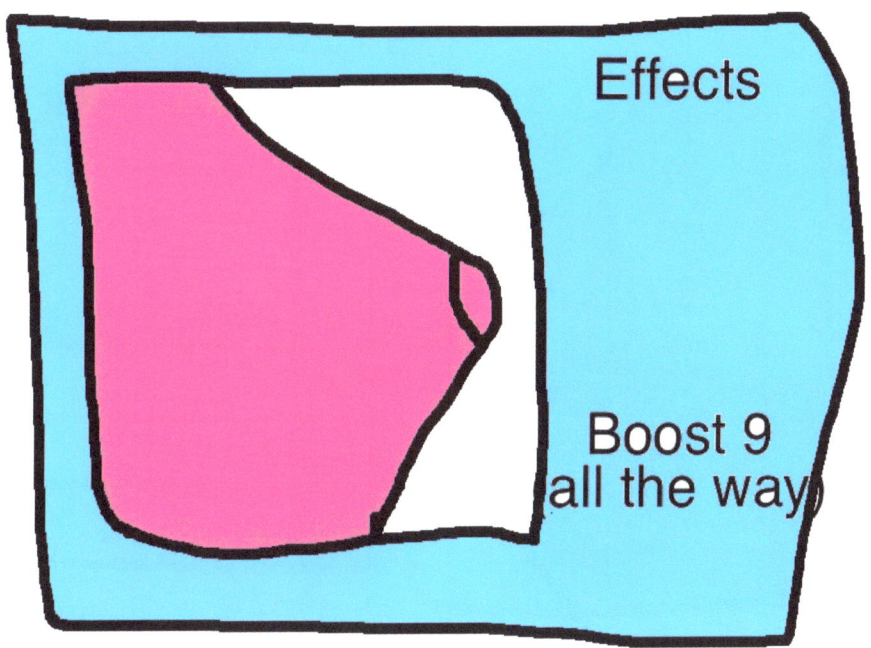

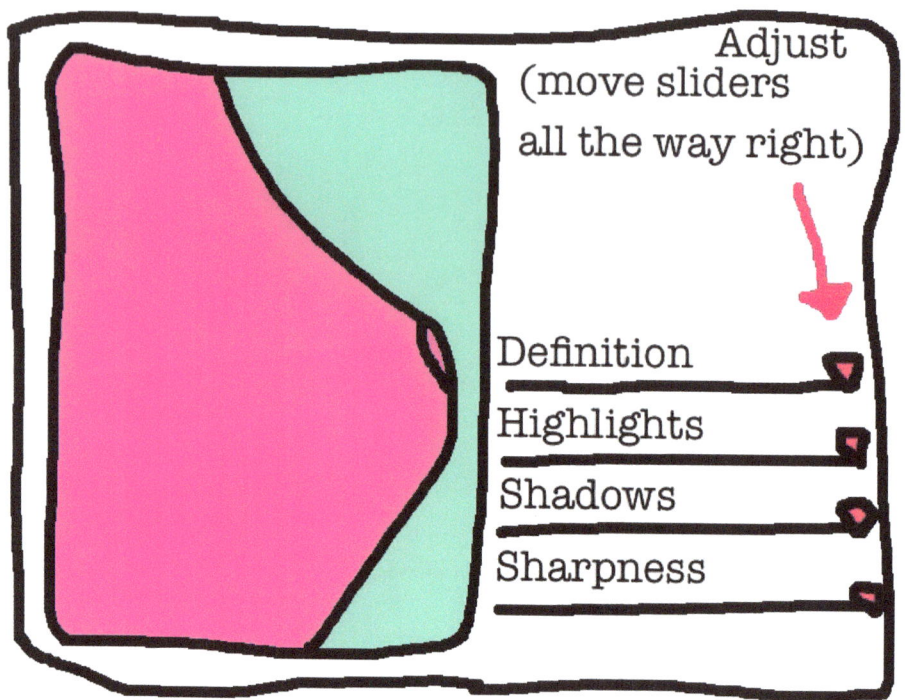

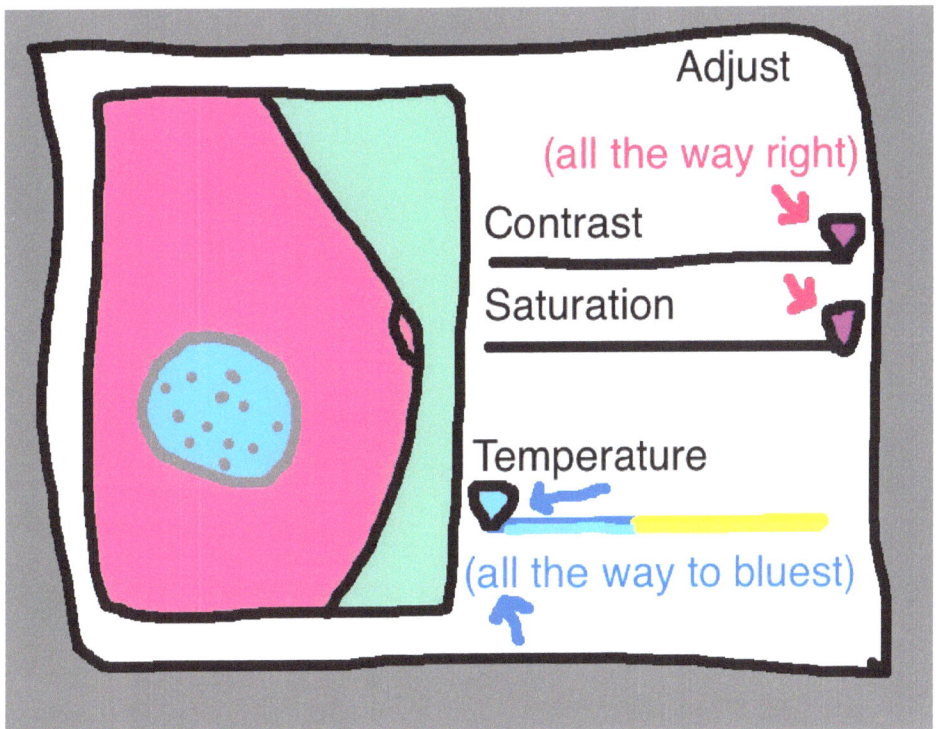

http://vimeo.com/110921987 This link takes you to our Vimeo video account, with a slightly longer DIY Mammogram movie that includes REAL screencaptures of how to do the editing correctly to see the lump under your skin...or watch it here...
[vimeo http://vimeo.com/110921987]

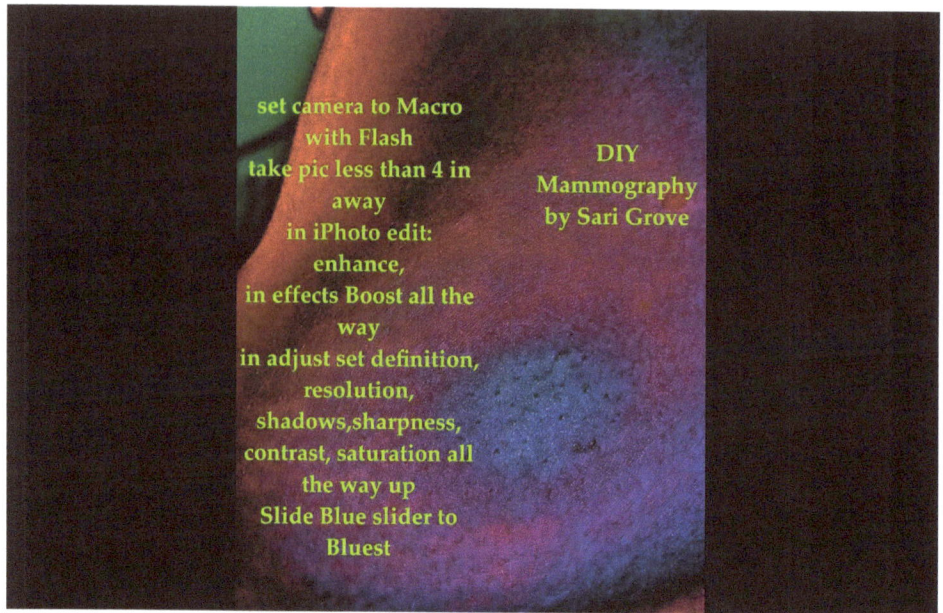

set camera to Macro with Flash take pic less than 4 in away in iPhoto edit: enhance, in effects Boost all the way in adjust set definition, resolution, shadows,sharpness, contrast, saturation all the way up Slide Blue slider to Bluest

DIY Mammography by Sari Grove

How to get the Iodine you need to shrink your breast lump...

Yup, it's going to get weird...
You need Iodine to shrink your breast lump...
Iodine is the element in the Adrenal Gland that antidotes Calcium...
Calcium is what is the base of the lump...Calcium excess in the Adrenal Gland is how you get lumps...Most Calcium excesses today are caused by taking some

form of a birth control drug, many many
years ago & it did not excrete...
Actually it is normal that it didn't
excrete...You have to force it out...

So even if you took birth control pills in your
20s & you are now 48, you still have a
calcium excess in your Adrenal Gland that
could create problems like a breast lump...

In fact, just before menopause is when
those lumps show up...

But it was so long ago that you took birth
control drugs, it couldn't possibly be
connected?

Think again...

Children born of mothers who took birth
control drugs inherit the Calcium excess...

Calcium excess in extreme causes Adrenal Gland failure...
Adrenal Gland failure is Aids...That simple...

On a milder level, Calcium excess just causes things like Gender Dysphoria...Girls feel like they are boys & vice versa...It's actually a biochemical tendency...

Ok...So anyways...My previous books talk about this stuff more, this is just about food & I am getting way too serious...

Please read the other books if you have queries...
(The Grove Health Science series is in order btw...)

Anyways...The pictures below show
 1)Dry Sea vegetables
2)Wet sea vegetables(you soak them for 7 minutes in cold water to rehydrate them)-

Oh big important-when "draining" the sea vegetables, grab them with your hand in a clump from the waterlogged bowl & plop them into another dry bowl...If you just tip the bowl sideways to drain out the excess water, you get the really really strong seaweed taste that is in the water & omigosh it's wow yucky...

 3)The package so you can know what it is in the store

So this sea vegetable salad contains Wakame, Agar, Suginori, & Tsunomata...Oh & Mafunori!

Translation:A whole lotta IODINE!!!

You serve it with some sliced apple pieces, some sliced onion pieces & some Japanese vinaigrette(usually rice vinegar, sesame oil, soy sauce with maybe some minced garlic or ginger)...(I put some Dijon horseradish mustard in the salad too, to lower that seaweed taste a bit!)

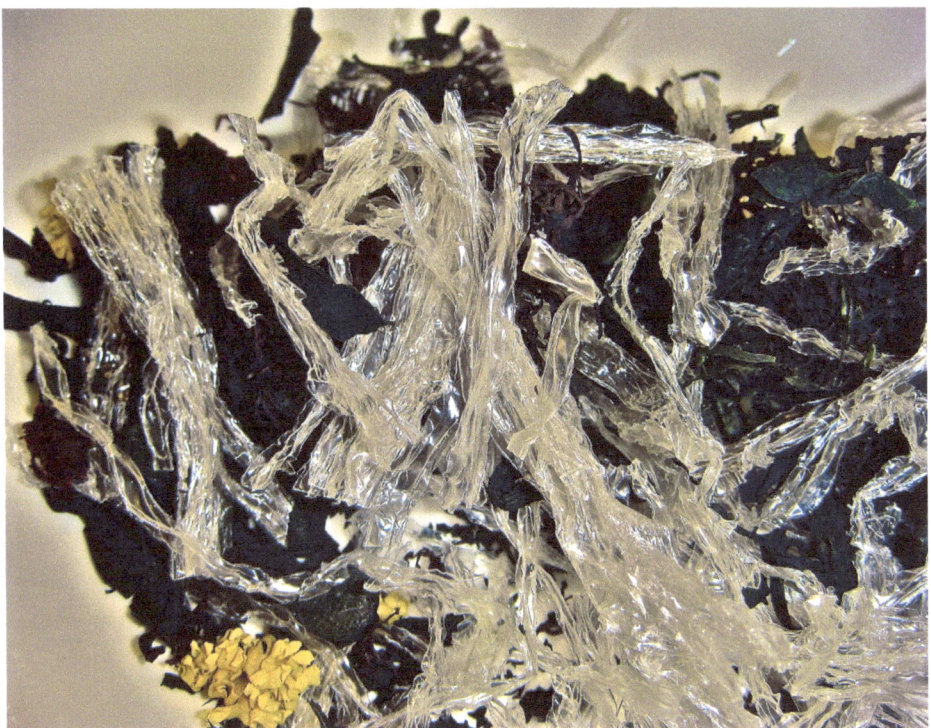

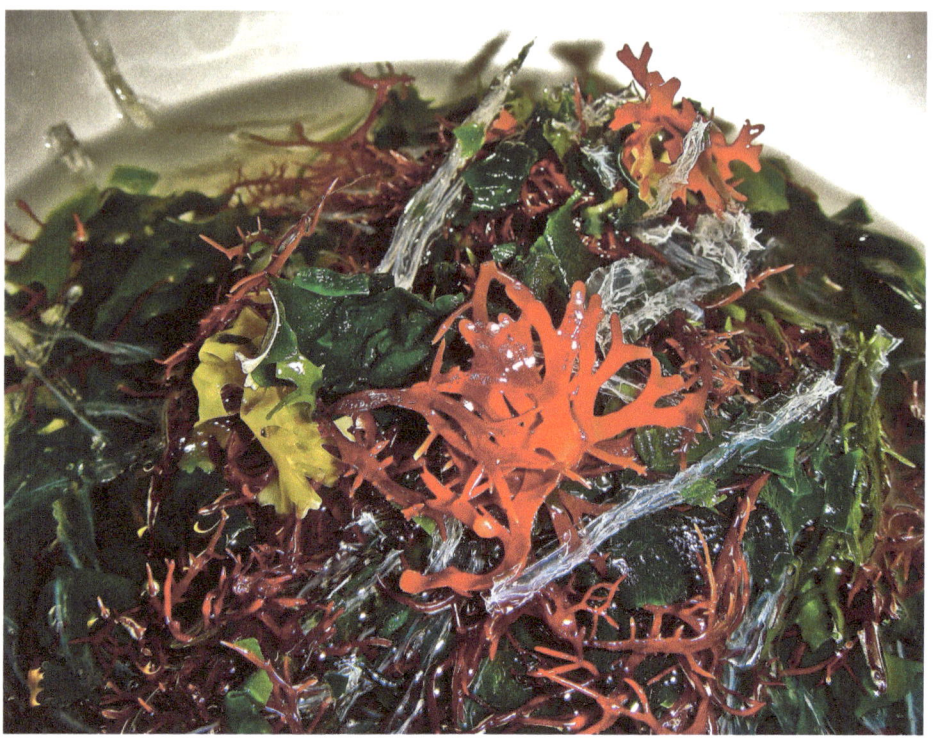

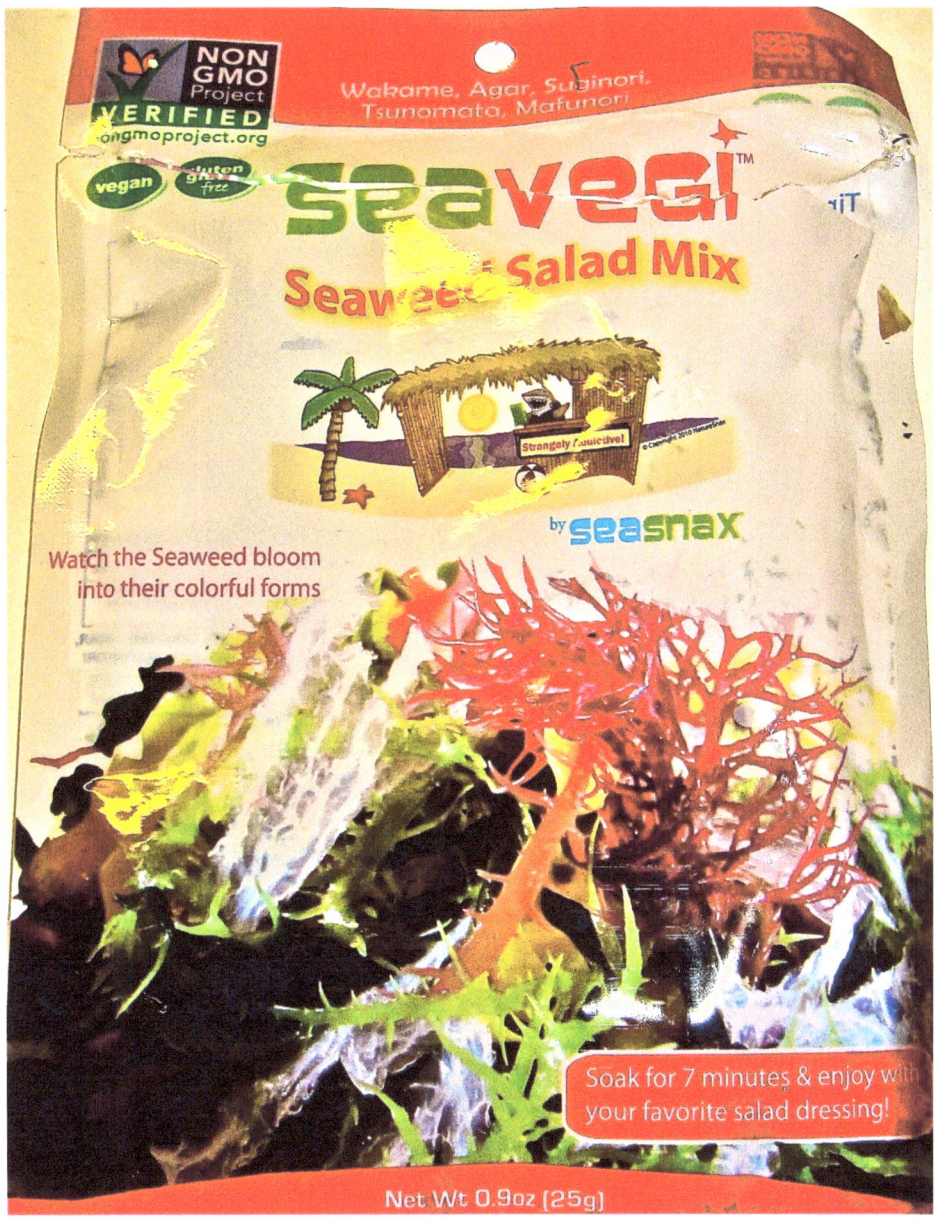

I'm an artist who innovates in the Medical Arts...

The writing of books happened because I needed a way to explain a new way of looking at medicine, & after a year of learning Blender 3d animation software, I decided a book was easier to make than an animated film!

My medical theory is actually a chart-the Grove Body Part Chart...

Organ	Minus element	Plus element
Thyroid	Zinc	Lead
Thymus	Manganese	Iron
Lungs Lymph Nodes	Titanium	Aluminum
Heart	Potassium	Aurum
Kidneys	Carbon	Nitrogen
Pancreas	Selenium	Sulphur
Liver	Oxygen	Hydrogen
Adrenal	Iodine	Calcium
Spleen	Copper	Phosphorus
Gallbladder	Magnesium	Mercury
Colon	Fluorine	Bismuth

The chart shows 11 body parts, & in each body part there are 2 elements that live together as opposites...

For example, in the Thyroid Gland there is Zinc & Lead...

Zinc is found in sunshine things like Vitamin D3...

Lead is found in potatoes & carrots...

Th elements are also divided as Minus elements or Plus elements...

Minus is a detoxifier, Plus is a nutrifier...

So Zinc detoxifies & Lead nutrifies...

This simplifies the body & disease...

Too much Zinc for example can cause Bipolar symptoms...

Too much Lead can cause Multiple Sclerosis symptoms...

If you have one or the other, you can use its OPPOSITE element as your medicine...

Our(my husband Joseph Grove is the "our"), first book is the Grove Body Part Chart:A Medical Arts Innovation...

Then we went on & wrote 5 more books which we then decided to call that series the Grove Health Science series...

RepoWoman is a nonsurgical breast cancer lump removal protocol...

It includes DIY Chemo, DIY Mammogram, & an exercise & diet recommendation...

RepoWoman is Book 6 of the Grove Health Science Series of Books, & stands on the shoulders & research of those earlier books...

(but unlike the other books in the series, RepoWoman just gives answers...

It is short enough to give as a gift to someone who has a breast lump

(or to yourself)

& is still in those very early stages of trying to get rid of it,

trying to avoid the

whole lumpectomy, radiation, chemotherapy, tamoxifen, regime...)

Women today are kicking & screaming to somehow get out of the breast cancer

regime trap...

Somehow, if they could only get rid of the breast lump somehow themselves,

the nightmare could end...

I am the author of this book, Sari Grove, & I myself faced this conundrum...

I faced the screaming throngs who said I would die if I didn't get surgery...

And so on...

I was in the middle of writing my 3rd book, & as it happens that book was about

avoiding surgery if you possibly could...

Determined to NOT be a hypocrite, I decided I was going to fix this lump thing

myself...

I was forced into the whole Mammogram, Ultrasound, Needle Biopsy,

Oncologist appointment ritual...

After getting the worst service possible, I knew I was finished...

I was going to solve breast cancer...I wasn't going back...

Book 3 got written...At the very end, I discover just how to reverse a malignant

lump to benign...

Not get rid of the lump...Just change the chemistry of it...It was a huge

breakthrough...It bought me time...A benign lump can sit for years...A malignant

lump is dangerous...

Book 4 I started trying to figure out how to get rid of the lump itself...

In Book 5 I start to nail down a protocol...

You realize this is all happening in the present, I am writing the books, & taking

pictures & taking my medicines...All at the same time...I am now on a raw plant

based diet...I have been walking 10 km(6 miles) almost every day...

Book 6 is RepoWoman...The protocol I came to after all the research &

practice...RepoWoman is just that...The answers I figured out...

I am still walking the 10 km every other day & am still leaning towards the plant

based raw diet & I still do the DIY Mammogram to check things & I still take a

much lower dosage of my DIY chemo to be careful...

But I have successfully avoided the lumpectomy protocol & whatever else they

had in store for me...

I am healthier than I have ever been, & happen to be 36 pounds lighter(by accident, the raw plant diet did this-no dieting)...

The best thing is, is that I UNDERSTAND what the lump chemistry is & I

UNDERSTAND how to deal with it...

I have my own science to back me up...

I have changed & corrected my own biochemistry, & I am in control of my life

like never before...

Instead of feeling disfigured & wounded by surgery, I feel gorgeous & sexy

because I have fought hard for this win...

CAUTIONARY WORDS:Being a RepoWoman is hard...It is a full time job...It is only for the brave...Be forewarned...A RepoWoman is a pioneer...Only the bold need apply...

Joseph Grove

Joseph Grove holds a double honours Bachelor of Arts in Philosophy & Comparative Literature from the University of Toronto...
Joseph's grandfather was a soldier who served in World War 1 in France, then went to Oxford on a Rhodes scholarship, & became a physician, then later served in WW2 as a doctor(In Halifax, Nova Scotia)...
Joseph married Sari on December 11, 1996, & they have now been married for almost 18 years...
Sari's father was a neuro-opthalmological surgeon & professor of medicine(as well as an author of several medical books & the

widely used textbook The Ophthalmic Assistant)...

Together, the pair(Joseph & Sari) found a synchronicity in being able to talk about & understand complex medical ideas...

Careerwise, it turned out that the arts were the most freeing in terms of allowing for innovation...

Joseph & Sari Grove became artists who innovate in the Medical Arts...

Hints on how to figure out what is in the drugs you are taking, & where they fit in on the Grove Body Part Chart, which will help you to know what they do to your body, so you can antidote them or prevent getting addicted to the drug...

Ok, so you are faced with a new drug name...You don't know what is in it exactly...So, I go to the wikipedia page for that drug name(or its generic equivalent page-wikipedia will tell you that...)

For example, I have never taken dramamine but I know someone who uses it for stomach flu(which is usually some sort of food poisoning)...

Interested, I checked the ingredients for dramamine in wikipedia...

Ok, so there seems to be 2 basic elements...(Long words & complicated looking)...

The first long word tells me what that ingredient does...Hmm...It seems to have sedative effects...Ha! I know that! Sedative type things are a TITANIUM element...On the Grove Chart, Titanium is in the Lung Lymph Node system...Ok, I know how Titaniums behave...Titaniums are painkillers, Titaniums lower cholesterol levels(cholesterol by the way is an Aluminum on our chart-the opposite element to Titanium, so that all makes sense)...Titaniums also have the unique effect of causing constipation...It's actually because Titaniums cause muscle weakness, so your muscles don't feel able to poop, but anyways the effect is constipatory...(Aluminums like Arnica for instance cause muscle strength, which is why athletes often take them)...Titaniums also cause memory loss, pretty quickly...Aspirin, Marijuana, Statins, Mint, Chamomile tea, Hulled Hemp seeds, are all Titaniums, just different titrations or dosages...

Ok so the first ingredient in the dramamine is a Titanium & works by stopping the diarrhea & the vomiting by causing muscle weakness(that constipatory effect)...Plus you have painkilling & sedation...

Let's look at the second ingredient in Dramamine...Oh this is going to be also pretty easy...It says the second ingredient is in the same family as Caffeine or Theobromine...I know Caffeine is a Copper, so number 2 ingredient is a Copper...Now the wikipedia on dramamine says the makers of the drug put the Copper thing into it because they were trying to offset the sedative effects of the first ingredient (because Copper makes you awake)...

But also, what isn't mentioned is that Copper things kill Salmonella things...So that is neat...

Now we know that dramamine is a Titanium & a Copper...So say maybe you were a more "natural" type person, & you had food poisoning & wanted to copy the drug in a more natural way...Ok, so just seek out a Titanium & a Copper & eat them together...Um, thinking caps on...How about you eat some hulled hemp seeds(Titanium)

& drink a really strong cup of black tea (Copper)?

The flow of elements...

Our Chart flows from top to bottom...It starts with the Thyroid & works its way down to the Colon at the bottom of the body parts... Now if we look closer, we are going to say that the flow of the elements INSIDE each body part, STARTS with the Minus element & follows with the Plus element...
Why am I saying this?
Well...I was thinking about a very very common substance...

Salt...

Salt is actually made up of 2 elements...The code for Salt is NaCl...So Na...& Cl...Na stands for Sodium...Cl stands for Chlorine... (You can find out what element codes stand for by checking the Periodic Table of

Elements-there are excellent versions online which tell you what is what & about each what too)...

Now Sodium is in the Mercury family, which on our Chart, is in the Gallbladder section as a Plus nutrifying element...

Chlorine is in the next body part down the chart, the Colon...Chlorine is in the Fluorine family...(many elements on the Periodic table are in the same family but much stronger than, or much weaker than, so they get their own name...)

Chlorine is a little weaker than Fluorine, but same effects...

We know Fluorine is antidoted by Bismuth Bi(charcoal)...If you check Chlorine gas for example you will notice that a gas mask with charcoal inside will protect you from chlorine fumes...That's a big hint that Fluorine & Chlorine act the same...Birds of a feather...

Now if Sodium Chloride, Salt, is a very common substance, that occurs readily, naturally, then...

Then we can see on the Chart that Sodium is the second element, the Plus element, in the Gallbladder, & that, Chlorine, in the Fluorine family, is the first element, a Minus element, in the very next body part down the chart...

So now we are going to theorize that a common natural substance on this earth, is starting with the Plus element of one organ, & connecting with its neighbour below it, the Minus element in the next body part, the Minus element...

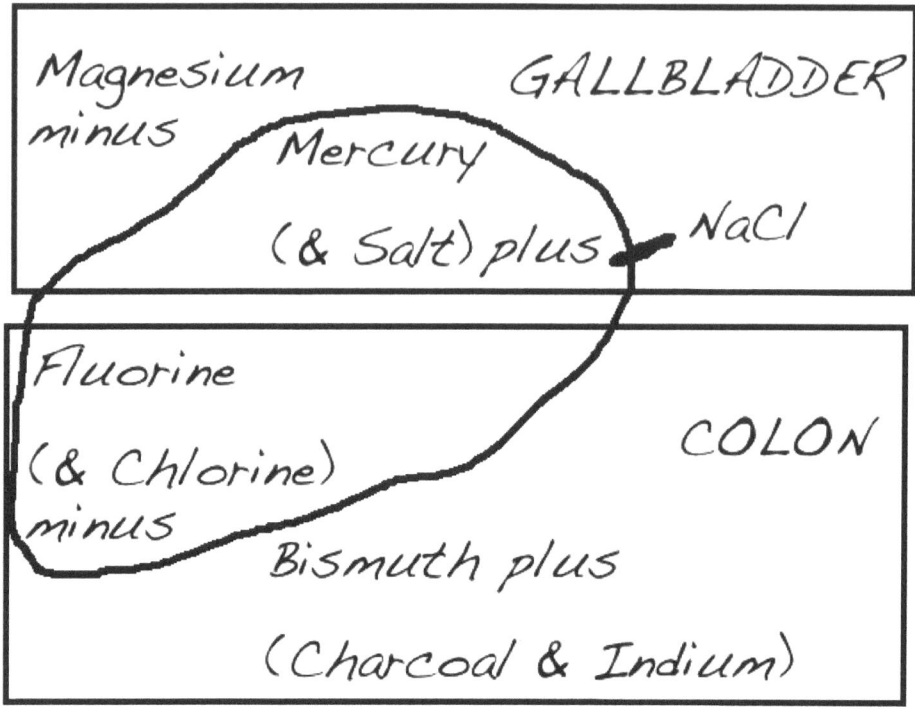

Magnesium minus

GALLBLADDER

Mercury

(& Salt) plus — NaCl

Fluorine

(& Chlorine) minus

COLON

Bismuth plus

(Charcoal & Indium)

By seeing how elements flow through the body parts(using our Chart as the guide), we can now know more about the flow of the body...

Let's try & see if we can duplicate this flow idea with another substance...

Water...

Hmm...How about water? That's pretty common...
Water in chemistry is written H_2O...That means Hydrogen 2, & one molecule of Oxygen...

Does that jibe with our theory of flow?

Umm...

Hydrogen is the Plus element in the Liver...

Oxygen is the Minus element...

Darn...

In water, the Plus element comes first, then the Minus element comes second...

Unless maybe in reality the Oxygen molecule showed up first, then bonded AFTER with the two Hydrogens?
Did chemists just write it backwards for convenience sake?

How do we know, or how could we find out which element ACTUALLY comes first in the FLOW of things?

When making water, did Oxygen actually come before the Hydrogen part?

Hmmm...Ok well...

Scientists pretty much say Hydrogen came first...

Helium next, which by the way is in the Oxygen family...

Then Oxygen...

So pretty probably, Hydrogen existed, then there was a catalyst, like a fire, or explosion sort of thing, which caused the Hydrogen to bond to its new friend, Oxygen, forming water...
In order to get Hydrogen to mate with Oxygen to form water you need some sort of spark or fire or explosion...Then you get water, H_2O...

If our bodies are mimetic copies of the universe, in material & flow & order, then probably Hydrogen should come before Oxygen in our own internal flow of things...Plus element(H) before Minus element(O)...

So now we have contradicted our Salt theory...Darn...

Could we try with something else? Hmm...

No, but wait! Salt occurs pretty naturally, but water require a catalyst...Does the necessity of the catalyst indicate that to create the water molecule that there needs to be a REVERSAL of atoms to get to water?

Then our Minus flowing to Plus element theory in the body might work...Hmmm...

Around December 2012, I drew this picture to try to explain how the elements on our chart would combine with each other to form the next element on the list...

So in the picture I drew Zinc as sunshine, combining with a Lead pencil in the Thyroid, to form the next element in the next body part, Iron...

Then I drew the Iron bar meeting up with a Manganese peanut in the Thymus, & forming Aluminum(a sheet of aluminum)...

Then that Aluminum sheet marries Titanium in the Lungs & Lymph nodes, & forms Aurum in the Heart...

I obviously got tired at that point, & left the rest of the flow as a 'to be continued'...

But I think the point was made...The body begins say with 2 elements, then they together create a third next element, which requires its mate, to form another & so on...

Unfortunately, even back then, I had not solidified which element, the Minus or the Plus came first...

So we are stuck on flow...

We know Lithium is in the same family as Lead...We know Lithium is one of the early earth elements...

So...

Did sunshine(Zinc) precede Lead (Lithium)???

Or... did Lithium(Lead family) come before sunshine(Zinc)...?

I was hoping to figure this out, but I am guessing this will have to be a subject that I will come back to when I have an "aha!" moment...

Feel feel to write me at grove@sent.com if you have a theory about which came first...

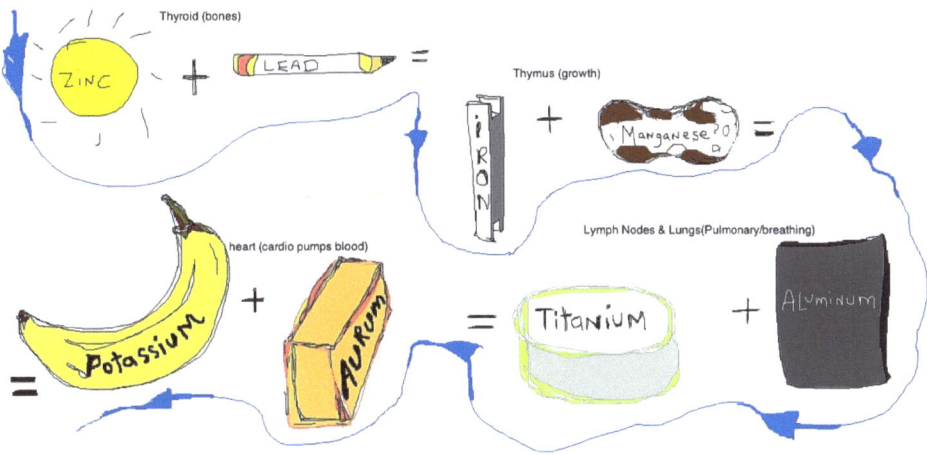

Chicken or Egg

On the subject of which came first, I should mention my own theory of chicken or egg...

My feeling is, is that God wrote the Holy Bible in order...(God through people's hands)...

So He starts with the Heavens & the Earth...

Then he moves on to more specific things like plants...

Then animals...

Then humans...

Which is pretty much the same thing as the theory of Evolution...

Eggs came before chickens...

Both God & science agree...

So my opinion is, is that the theory of Creation & the theory of Evolution are in agreement...No fight...No argument...

The main difference for me is that one gives credit to God & the other doesn't as much...

But one could say that Evolutionists could believe in God creating stuff, they just aren't mentioning it overtly...

As an artist who creates things, I like to get credit...

So personally I go with the theory of the Creation version, mainly because it gives credit...

I like to err on the side of caution...If God created all these things, then I'd better give credit...

Because if I don't give credit, & I am wrong not to, then I have a pretty powerful upset Artist who is now mad at me...

Very short religious bio...

I became a Christian in 1987 while attending McGill University...I was Jewish up until the age 21, became a Christian, & now at this writing, I have been a Christian for 27 years...(Yes I am 48 now)... Joseph is United Church...A more "normal" upbringing, no big change except for marrying me (who still carried some very very different cultural habits)...

In the Brain...

If you remove the Hypothalamus, which is the Phosphorus producing centre which produces Phosphorus(testosterone?)in the Spleen...

Then...

The PAIRED brain part, the Globus Pallidus, which produces the Copper element for the Spleen, becomes DOMINANT...

So, by removing the Hypothalamus you get Minus element Copper dominance in the brain & in the Spleen...

If you radiate the Hypothalamus, (radiation providing a Minus element ray like a Zinc or Gamma ray say), then also, testosterone or Phosphorus should be lowered in the Hypothalamus...

HOWEVER if you DAMAGE the Hypothalamus or the Spleen, you will get a BUILDUP of Phosphorus...

Too much Phosphorus can be seen in Parkinson's disease...

IN GENERAL, Damage to a body part creates an EXCESS of the Plus element...

REMOVING a body part however creates a MINUS element dominance...

For example, removing a Gallbladder causes long term symptoms of MAGNESIUM excess(the Minus element)- like poohing too much...

But a damaged Gallbladder causes symptoms of excess mercury, the Plus element...Excess Mercury is high Bilirubin levels, & can manifest as jaundice, stuttering, Tourette's syndrome, dyslexia or autism ADHD disorders...

Radiating organs is adding a Minus element like a Zinc ray...So that should LOWER the Plus element in excess...

So radiating the body(suntanning beds) should lower Calcium excess in the Adrenal Gland...Calcium excess is a precursor to

cancer & a few other serious problems...
(which is why I think sunshine & radiation &
tanning beds are useful medicinally in any
form of cancer therapy...My take is that all a
suntanning bed does is force Calcium
excess out of your body to rise to the
surface...In takes it away from core vital
body parts...The blobs of calcium or even
Phosphorus appear on your skin because
the suntanning forces it out to the
surface...The body protects & detoxifies by
forcing bad things to the outside...So
suntanning does NOT cause skin cancer-it
merely forces the Calcium & Phosphorus
out of your Adrenal Gland & up to your
skin's surface...seeing those blobs may be
scary, but it is even scarier to have Calcium
excess living invisibly inside your body
where you cannot see it & it can spread
silently...)
P.S. Licorice Root extract applied topically
to those blobs does wonders in getting rid

of them...Licorice root is a strong Copper that eats Phosphorus mold...

p.p.s.Yogurt & other so-called probiotics substances are in the fermented Phosphorus category & I think they are entirely the absolutely WRONG thing to eat if you are worried about Calcium excess, Cancer or even Parkinson's disease...

Mustard Gas

Did you know mustard gas was first used as a war weapon? Long story short, it was discovered that inhaling the gas, (kind of like inhaling Garlic, a Selenium element on our chart-mustard is also a Selenium element, as is cayenne pepper...) lowered white blood cell counts? Selenium things lower blood sugar in the Pancreas actually...Which is why eating Cayenne pepper with your food can help prevent diabetes(or even reverse)...

Anyways...Mustard Gas as a weapon lead to the very first forays into chemotherapy against Cancer...Cancer is a calcium excess combined with a Phosphorus excess in the Spleen, & an iron excess in the Thymus gland...Some tumors feed on Sulphur otherwise known as Sugar, so Mustard gas, being a Selenium would lower Sulphur Sugar levels, thus starving a tumor that had alot of Sulphur Sugar inside... (Tumors are very dependent on what you eat yourself, which is why they are so unique to your eating habits...)
Truth is, white blood cells are up in the Thymus gland, they are the Manganese thing there...Iron is the red blood cell...But still, they were onto something...

What weapon that is used today could be converted into something that saves lives instead?

Or are weapons necessary in this world to get rid of bad people? Is it wrong to try to beat your sword into a plough? Are we in the "last Days" when it is time for bad people to pay their dues?
Is the peacemaking time way over?

Um...

The chemicals used in older fashioned photographic processing can have a tendency to produce Lung Cancer...For example, Aluminum Chloride, a hardener (at the end of the fixing process for printing), has an affinity to clog up the Lungs & Lymph node system...

(from my blog)(a R.I.P. article)
SARI GROVE (SARIGROVE.COM)

SOMEONE TOLD ME ABOUT GICLEES & I THOUGHT IT WAS A SURE THING!(WARNING:SAD ARTICLE)

NOVEMBER 10, 2014 | GROVECANADA

After universities & colleges & travel & such, I started painting because the sunset views from my apartment were so spectacular…

The sky was a miasma of fluffy orangey clouds with a purple note or green tinge…

My Dad said I should be a career painter…

So, I decided to listen, because that was the first career advice my Dad had ever given me…

I painted in oils in my bedroom at my parent's house, until one day, with oil paint left in a square shape from the edges, adorned my pretty quilt, I decided it was time to rent a studio…

Down at Sherbourne south of Front was a giant purple building where my studio was, & down the hall was a recording studio & up the stairs were a bevy of other independent artists…

It was perfect for me at about 500 square feet for $500 dollars a month & I felt like a superstar…

I had a few studio shows & then I started showing in galleries…

One of the earliest was a new co-operative gallery & the ideamaker of that gallery was big on this new technology(at the time) called giclees printing, which used inkjet printers to spray the inks in a more painterly fashion than typical poster style photographic lithography…

Me, a fan of ZeitGeist, Spirit of the Time, thought it was worth a swirl, so I set about finding some good art photographers, because there was no way I could take a picture of my paintings myself…

At the time, it was between 1993 & 1995-ish as I remember, I was still struggling with film rolls & my Mum's gift of a camera, & dark winter light or indoor yellow light, & getting back rolls where half the pictures were overexposed or flash burnt or unusable because colours were off or too dark to see…

Lord I think God invented digital cameras just for me I was so frustrated…

Anyways, I somehow found out that the best of the best art photographers were this company called "See Spot Run"…

Their then studio wasn't too far for me, also at the bottom of the city, & I went after calling & got to chat for a while with Noel who was the chattier one of two…

Two meaning yes there were two, twins, brothers who worked together, & I did my very best to stare & stare & stare & listen so that on future meetings I would have already figured out who was who by subtle differences…

I decided to identify Noel as the more friendly salesy one, & David was more the serious artistic one…Boy they really did look alike but soon I thought they were completely different just by tuning into their personalities…

Noel handled the business side of things then & David was more mysterious & took the pictures…

Of course the work was unbelievable good & my work looked so much better in the photographs, actually it was a giant transparency they made for me, that we then mailed to Altron Colour Imaging in New Brunswick who were the first in Canada to do this giclees thing…

I remember Noel telling off the Altron people because they said there wasn't some sort of bar chart or something technical that Altron needed to calibrate their inkjet printers & computers to…

Noel was saying:"Professionals USE THEIR EYES, not a chart…" He won over the phone & Altron got the work done…

Beautiful work by the way too, the fresh air of New Brunswick again added a new dimension to my paintings…

The giclees were mailed back to me & the work looked 10 times better than the original paintings…

When I showed them at the co-op gallery finally, I looked like a really great artist…I think at the time it helped me to believe that I was really good, despite the fact that the real work had been done by Noel & David & Altron…

But the confidence I got from working with real pros was worth every penny…Back then one picture, just one picture of one painting could cost you maybe $150.00 …

Back then you were grateful…These days people take 1000 pictures themselves with their own digital cameras & professional photographers often don't even get into the mix…

It is sad because working with a real pro is such a learning experience for a young artist…Of course Noel & David were working with film too…Real cameras…Real lights…Real studio…It was all real…

I write this post today because I just found out, 2 years ago, that Noel & David died… Yes, died…Both…

I am a little in shock…

David Saltmarche apparently around January 2011, & Noel Saltmarche about 2 months later in March of 2011…

I am a little shocked…Oh, did I say that already? They were both only about 61 years old…

One of the obits online mentions donations for David could go to Princess Margaret to benefit Lung Cancer research so I guess it was lung cancer…

Around 2004, I was sort of getting famous as an artist & I was showing some very big painting in a giant gallery in Hazelton Lanes…

I had a wonderful Picasso-esque in feel watercolour with oil pastel piece of my brother's Bernese Mountain Dog, & it was already framed by Yorkville Fine Frame in expensive but low key looking gold leaf & plexiglass…

I decided to look up See Spot Run again & do a giclees run because the painting was so iconic…Plus watercolours fade so I thought I could save it a bit that way…For time…

I brought the work to Carlaw, a newer location & Noel was there & welcomed me & we chatted & now See Spot Run was doing giclees printing in house & I said ok & that was that…Said hi to David in passing he was always so busy…

They had just done the catalogue for Cy Twombly & I was so impressed…

Noel showed me work for the Hudson's Bay company…The artist Erica Shuttleworth was there since she was showing with Drabinsky I think…

I left & went to the Hazelton gallery & told the owner about my plans AND…

He totally freaked…Freaked…I don't know if it was graven images or mechanical printing or giclees are crap or what, but I had done something very very very wrong…

OMIGOSH big mistake…Ordering this work was a big mistake…The gallery owner was so mad at me…

I called Noel & told him what had happened…He said:"David already took the picture"…

Oh no…

I was still shell-shocked from being screamed at by my gallery…

I went into paralysis mode…I did nothing…I didn't go to pay for the work done…I didn't

go to pick my painting up…I didn't do
anything…
I just did nothing…I hoped my mistake
would slowly just go away, just get
enveloped in a giant cloud like
you see in paintings…
Time passed…Eventually the Hazelton
gallery closed…I moved on to another
gallery & another & another…
Ever since 9/11 2001, the gallery business
was dicey & I knew that, so I kept moving
like a shark knowing if I stopped, well, I just
kept moving…
Somehow I always managed to get out in
time & land on my feet…I got better &
better…
So much time had passed that I now felt
guilty about the money I owed See Spot
Run for the photograph of my painting,
even though I never got to see it…
But so much time had passed I was now
too embarrassed to just show up with

money…It wasn't the money anyway, it was just I was still paralyzed because I knew if I had the transparency that I would probably still go ahead & make giclees, but that somehow that was wrong…

I couldn't pick up the slide because then I would follow through…By then I knew giclees were a bit dumb & a bit of a marketing thing & there wasn't really a windfall of cash or fame to be had in a giclees…

When I first had them done I sold a bunch because it was such a new thing & we were all enamoured of the new technology…But as time passed people got bored & learned that they were still a photograph & that the artist hadn't really done much to participate…It was still a machine made reproduction…

Artists learned the markups weren't great… Again, at that time there were initial start up costs for giclees…Also minimum orders…

Much more time passed…I phoned See Spot Run to explain my paralysis again more thoroughly, & David laughed…He chatted with me for such a long time on the phone, he talked about the ice glistening on the hay in a barn in the morning & the steam of a horse's nostrils & as he spoke I could see the crackly ice & feel the warm brood of the Mare & I knew he was a genius…

I used some of that phone conversation that year to formulate an artist statement I was working on…Once again I sounded so much deeper than I truly was, just from my brush with greatness…

Funny…David didn't ask me about the money owed & he didn't care when we hung up, friends, & I hadn't committed to coming by…I secretly was hoping they had a PayPal account so I could just email money without having to show up in person-I mean it was scandalous how many

years had gone by without me paying my
bill…

I don't even know how much it was for…
Maybe $150??? Wasn't sure…Too
embarrassed to ask…I'm not poor & had
never owed anyone money before…

In the back of my head I decided God
wanted me to gift my painting to them…The
Gold Leaf frame by itself was at least 500
dollars, which was alot at that time…The
painting was maybe the best of that
collection…It was really good…I decided
that it was nice that they had this painting…

I gift many paintings to people & I had not
gifted Noel & David ever…This was a
sneaky way of giving them a gift I thought…

I let it go…

Silly me…It's 2014 & someone was mean
to me in a new author's group I just
joined…Yes, I am writing books now…
About medicine…It turns out I have a knack
for thinking outside of the box, the artist

thing, but in particular I am really good at doing that when it comes to medical ideas…

My parents are a bit of a hybrid couple, so my knack makes sense…

So today, this Sunday in November, the 9th, 20014, the really rude lady in this author's group triggered the memory of that gallery owner screaming at me about giclees…

I thought of Noel & David & the painting…I wondered if they had a website yet, maybe they had a PayPal button I could just secretly send them $150 dollars without conversation…

As I typed in see Spot Run & Noel & David (not even knowing their last name because in the art world that is not important if you are friends with people who do good work), saw a weird comment about how "David WAS…"

My heart stopped…What did she mean by was???

was…was…was…What did was mean…
I found out their Dad was Ken Saltmarche
the head of the Art Gallery of Windsor…
Also a pretty famous artist…
Then I found out…
Both of these people, these 2 people I knew
myself, these two very good people, these
2 artists, these 2 twin brothers, these two
friends were no longer…
I am so sad I can barely cry & my throat is
dry & I don't know what to feel…
I thought I should call them at the number
at their studio to say I was going to come by
& then I realized again that if people were
no longer alive I could not call them…
It is like this with artists…Two ships passing
in the night kind of thing…We are all pretty
nomadic so we don't see each other
often…
I mean, we don't see our own friends…It's
not a job where you go to an office every

day & the same people are there for 15 years…

I often find out that artists have passed away, years after the fact, by internet accident…

I cry by myself & sometimes get in touch with the family or write about it or something…

I am writing about it now because that is what I can do now…

I am so sorry for your loss, my loss, to the sons & daughters & other friends & passerby & other clients & to the art world…

My grandfather & his brother were Lou & Nat Turofsky of Alexandra Studios & they were also photographers…

The founding collection of the Hockey Hall of Fame is made up of the Turofsky Collection…

You can see some of their works at this link http://www.hhof.com/htmlphotogalleries/gallery_turofsky001.shtml
(Legends of Hockey – Gallery – Lou & Nat Turofsky, 001
The Turofsky collection pictorially depicts two decades of the "original six" era featuring black and white player portraits and game action from the NHL.
www.hhof.com/htmlphotogalleries/gallery_turofsky001.shtml)
So, you see, 2 brothers, who were photographers, is a story very close to my heart…
I don't have any links to Noel & David's work because I couldn't find any online…
The work they did for me was before jpegs & pngs & digital cameras & I never converted that stuff to computer…
*If you type the name Ken Saltmarche into Google,(their father) you will get some really nice articles & even a catalogue of his

works as a pdf with some of the other artworks the family collected in the catalogue…

Thank you for listening to me…I feel a little better for writing this…

I hope Noel or David's children have kept the painting that I left in the See Spot Run studio & I hope it eases their grief a little to have it…

My love to the Saltmarche family who I don't really know but I know because I knew Noel & David & the apple cannot fall far from that darned tree…

If you ever need $150 bucks, call me…I owe you…

Sari

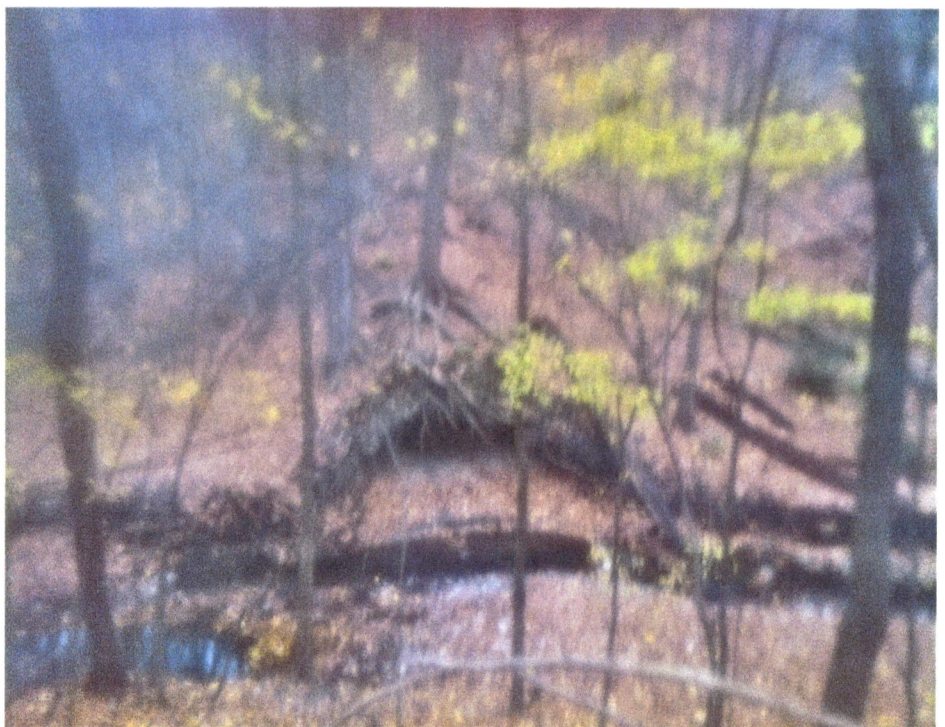

Picture shows a tree's root system on a little hilly area,

where underneath a little cave has formed, which enters into the river...I was imagining living in that little cave under the tree's roots, & venturing to the tiny beach to get water...(location:Moore Park Ravine, photo by Sari Grove using gold colour iPhone 4S...)

Cycling...Hitting your head with hemet on...Concussion...After effects...Let's look at one possibility angle of impact & how it could affect the human...

I am in the middle of reading Detour
(**Detour**
Cycling, coma and living with a brain injury
by Nick Mercer),

 but had to stop because I have some input...My 7th book deals with the brain, but it is based on work from earlier books of mine...I am familiar with the bipolar symptoms upon collapse of the left side of the Frontal lobe-you get a Zinc excess & a lack of Lead Pb, like Lead you eat in potatoes or carrots...(So you could eat more of those types of things to boost your Lead & that left frontal lobe...)If the impact crossed in as deep as the Globus Pallidus which it looks like it did, that is a Copper producing area, so you will feel not as awake, because the Hypothalamus takes over with Phosphorus sleepy dominance...You can compensate for that, & try to rebuild that area by adding some Coppers to your diet like Coriander(also called Cilantro it is a salad type thing you can just eat like salad)...I say Cilantro because that Copper has an affinity for the brain...Other sources of Copper may not be as effective in getting up to there...Your book is wonderful thank you...Sari Grove

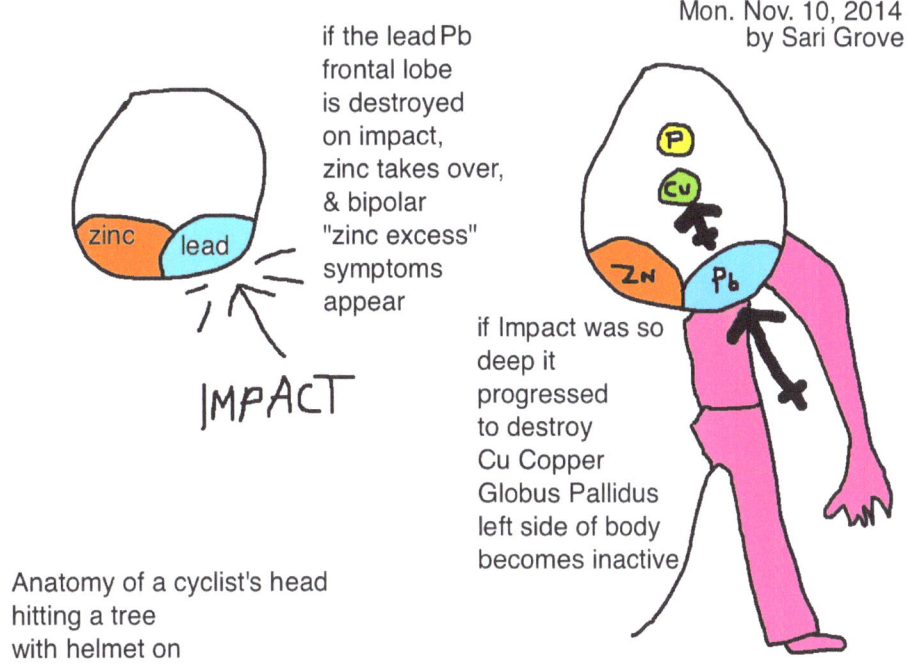

if the lead Pb
frontal lobe
is destroyed
on impact,
zinc takes over,
& bipolar
"zinc excess"
symptoms
appear

Mon. Nov. 10, 2014
by Sari Grove

IMPACT

if Impact was so
deep it
progressed
to destroy
Cu Copper
Globus Pallidus
left side of body
becomes inactive

Anatomy of a cyclist's head
hitting a tree
with helmet on

Oh I forgot to add...Generally in most concussion, there is a rise in Potassium levels, with a commensurate drop of Aurum...

This affects the Medulla Oblongata which controls the heart...It is very important to boost Aurum levels post concussion...Aurum is found in Taurine things like clam juice...Boosting Taurine is vital...High Potassium is very very dangerous because your heart becomes enlarged but weak...So boost your taurine if you can-you can buy Taurine powder & stick it in your drinks to get more...It will prevent cardiomyopathy...

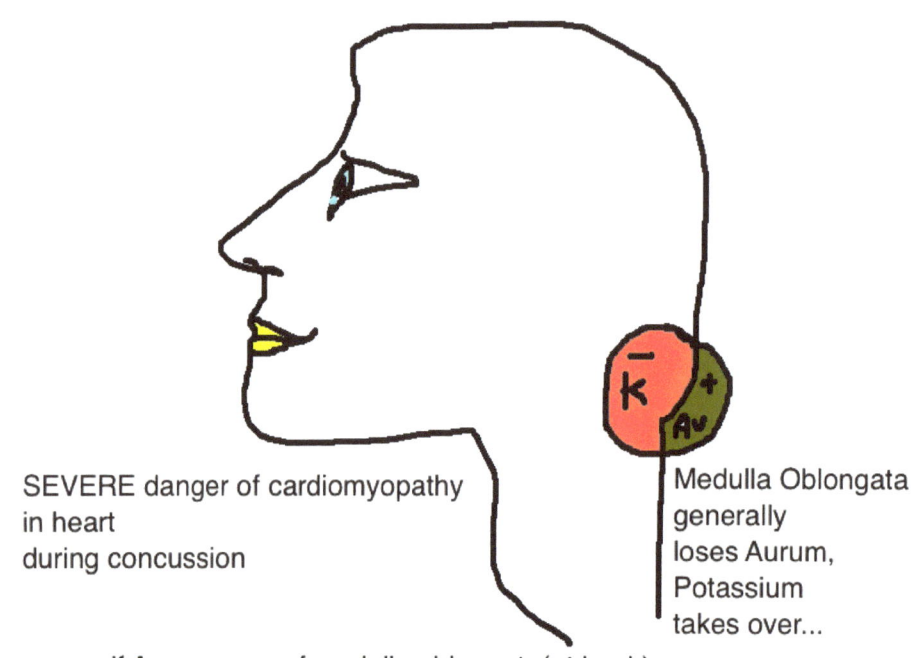

SEVERE danger of cardiomyopathy in heart during concussion

Medulla Oblongata generally loses Aurum, Potassium takes over...

if Aurum area of medulla oblongata(at back) fails, then Potassium dominance occurs

If the fall is to the back of the head, on the right side, the Selenium side, of the Occipital lobe(& that area fails), then you get Sulphur Sugar dominance in the Pancreas & eyes & of course that section of the Occipital Lobe...

FALL TO BACK OF HEAD
RIGHT SIDE

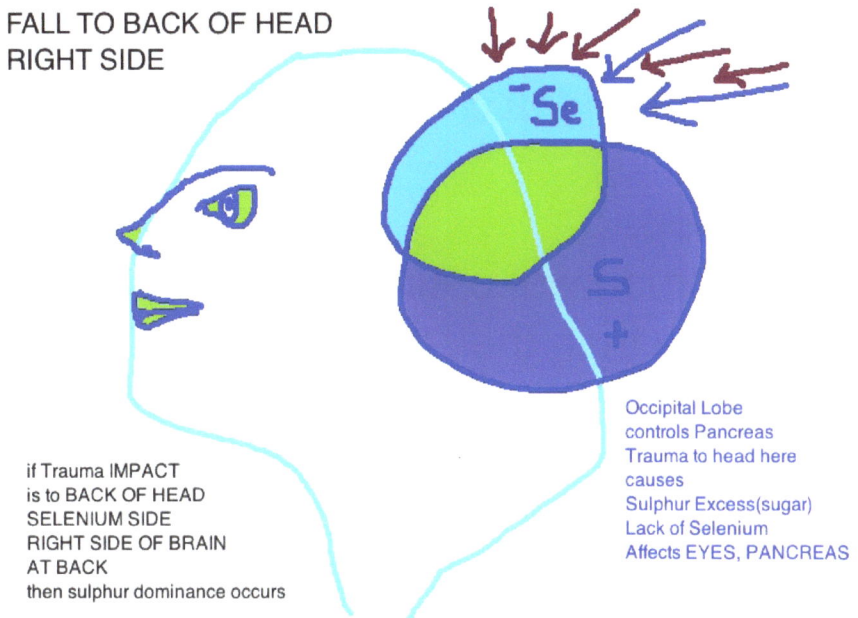

if Trauma IMPACT
is to BACK OF HEAD
SELENIUM SIDE
RIGHT SIDE OF BRAIN
AT BACK
then sulphur dominance occurs

Occipital Lobe
controls Pancreas
Trauma to head here
causes
Sulphur Excess(sugar)
Lack of Selenium
Affects EYES, PANCREAS

Revisiting the order of things...

But tea is so delicious with milk, they go so well together...Nature makes things delicious when it is the right order of things...

So let's look at tea & milk...

Milk is Calcium...

Tea is Copper...

To put it crudely of course...Both are so much more than their prime elements...

On the Grove Chart, The Adrenal Gland comes before the Spleen, & so Calcium comes before Copper...

If the Plus element of the Adrenal Gland, flows nicely & naturally into the Minus element, let's say the FIRST element of the Spleen, Copper, then we are confirming our early theory that the Plus element is the Second element in the order of things in the body parts...

We got screwed up with the idea of water, because water seems to be backwards...But then we remembered that water requires an explosion of sorts to get those elements to marry...Which probably indicates a reversal...

I mean, if you needed an explosion to get 2 people to marry each other, that might indicate it was not a natural thing, a natural order...

So if tea & milk are happy together, & they marry easily, or just date well, then we are maybe confirming the thought that MINUS elements come BEFORE plus elements on the Chart, & in the FLOW of the Body Parts...

Remembrance Day, Veteran's Day, Armistice Day, Day of the Dead...

Crestor has another side effect besides memory loss...It can cause leg cramps...Let's look at that...

Statin drugs are Titaniums, in the Lung Lymph Node system...Titanium is a Minus element, the detoxifiers...Aluminum is its counterpart, sometimes known as cholesterol, found in eggs, Arnica, Agave, chocolate, concrete...

So Titanium removes Aluminum...

If a person with high cholesterol, Aluminum, takes Crestor Titanium, the Titanium MINUSES(as a verb) the cholesterol...

Cholsterol is found in MUSCLE tissue, the Lungs & Lymph Nodes are muscular...

So if you take TOO MUCH Crestor, you start to burn though muscle...

When you start burning through muscle tissue in your body, you can feel leg cramps...That's the muscles in your legs being dissolved by the Statin drug...

http://www.mayoclinic.org/diseases-conditions/high-blood-cholesterol/expert-answers/rhabdomyolysis/faq-20057817

The technical term is called RHABDOMYOLYSIS...(the link above takes you to a Mayo clinic explanation of that)...Leg cramps...You can also duplicate this burning of muscle effect, the leg cramp thing, by exercising too much without eating enough...So, theoretically, the cure for leg cramps would be to put some cholesterol back in your body, stop taking Crestor or whatever Statin you are taking(aspirin counts, as do asthma drugs), or stop exercising so much, or sit on a concrete rock or concrete chair to osmote the natural Aluminum there...

(information about leg cramps as side effect comes from Arlene the lady I met at the Bloor Street Market while discussing the merits of Mandarin oranges in the new red fishnet bags with the handles...)

Back to the order of things for a moment...

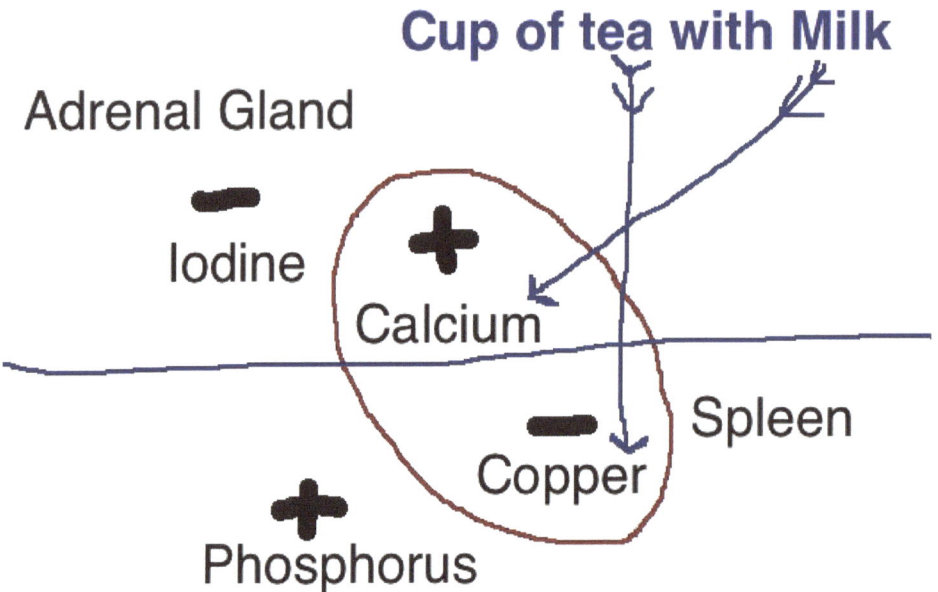

About chemistry...

So let's look at bread...Bread is some sort of grain mashed up, then you add some yeast to make it rise & be fluffy...
Grains are usually Nitrogens, the Plus element in the Kidneys...

Yeast, you would think, is a Phosphorus, maybe like cheese, or mold, but not in a bad mold way...
So Bread is Nitrogen & Phosphorus maybe...But I think you add Milk too, so that is Calcium, the Plus in the Adrenal Gland...Some people add a spot of sugr to make a bun sweet(Chinese bakery), so sugar is the Sulphur element, the Plus in the Pancreas...
If you add some water to mix the powders then you are adding a Hydrogen, the Plus in the Liver...But there is a little Oxygen in the water, which is the Minus element in the Liver...
Also, when you put it in the oven you add heat, which is Fire, & Fire is more Oxygen usually...Actually different levels of heat are different Minus elements on the Chart...At the top of the chart the Minus elements are weak & the Plus elements are strong...
(Opposites remember)...

So as you go down the chart, & the body parts, the Minuses get stronger & the Pluses get weaker...

So Zinc is a weak Minus element, but Fluorine is a very strong Minus element...

Lead is a very strong Plus element, bit looking to the last Plus element, at the bottom of the chart, Bismuth(charcoal) is a weak Plus element...

So a ray of sunshine, on a spring day might be Zinc temperature...But an electrical current at a acupuncturist's office might be Copper level strength-too hot, might burn a tendon!!!

So the temperature of the heat changes the Nature of the Minus element we will name it...

But for clarity, I like to think of FIRE as Oxygen, because that is in the middle of the list & is a good basic starting point...

A candlelight flame is probably like an Oxygen, that is where I am going from...Maybe 800 degrees celsius is the Oxygen temperature of a candle flame...

As a sidenote: There are now some metals that have a low burning threshold, so low that they are UNDER the 800 degree mark of a candle flame...

What that means is that say you want to do a little welding-join 2 pieces of metal together-you could get some low threshold burning metal & use a candle flame to melt it, & then use that sticky stuff to join up your 2 pieces of hard metal...(That is what welding is by the way-melting a metal that gets sticky & using that gluey metal to stick two other pieces of really hard metal together...The join is usually weaker, but it is still better than nothing...Of course, you could always use galvanized threaded metal rods & bolt them together using plumber's copper strapping as the joiner, by sticking the rods THROUGH the holes in the copper, bolting each rod in each hole, then that copper can be twisted a little in any direction to get your directional need-ie: perpendicular join or whatever...This works stronger than tying the metal rods together with wire because tying can slip whereas bolts are bolted...)

I noticed...
I noticed that after supplementing with Iodine(Madagascar periwinkle, Iodoral, Figwort, Nettle Leaf Tea, Poke Root, Kelp) that I lost my craving for sushi...
I also noticed that after supplementing with Licorice Root(Copper) that I lost my craving for Tea(copper)...
So if you are addicted to sushi(the Iodines), or addicted to coffee or tea(Coppers), you may have a serious nutritional deficiency in those areas that could be better addressed by a stronger dosage, or attention & awareness of that matter...

Alcohol is a heavy duty Hydrogen supplier...
If you are addicted to Alcohol, you may be getting Too much Oxygen somehow in your life...I know that sounds impossible thee days, too MUCH Oxygen???
But there are some athletes who are outdoors all the time, or soldiers on duty outside all the time...Or park rangers?
"Canadian Park Ranger rescue:"Come over here, get into my truck!"...
People who get way too much Oxygen are going to want to drink alot of Hydrogen things...Alcohol is like Heavy Hydrogen, way alot more of Hydrogen than water because the heaviness of distillation or just sitting around in an oak barrel causes the Oxygen to squish out or fume out...
End of this section Wed. Nov. 12, 2014 12:02 pm Eastern Standard Time...

Monday	Tuesday	Wednesday	Thursday
eat 'n drink	eat 'n drink	eat 'n drink	eat 'n drink
wash 'n dress	wash 'n dress	wash 'n dress	wash 'n dress
walk	walk	walk	walk
walk	walk	walk	walk
reward	reward	reward	reward
grocery shop	grocery shop	grocery shop	grocery shop

The RepoWoman suggested schedule idea plan...

Explanation: Wake up whenever you wake up naturally, no alarm clock or time constraints or guilt...Whenever you feel rested enough to get out of bed, that is when you begin...

Eat 'n drink means eat your raw salad vegetables with your oil & vinegar & lemon & the assorted nuts & some apple pieces if you feel sorry for yourself & need sweetness(so not all the time with the fruit thing)...Take your "medicines" ie your licorice root capsules, your black tea or coffee(cheat with a drop of milk but milk is a no no so really just enough to kill the acidity of the Copper in the caffeine)...If you want to take some of your herbs in tea form, be aware the Madagascar periwinkle makes you sleep, so now you will be in bed all day...Licorice root herb tea makes you awake so fine for mornings you are exercising...The Mugwort Artemisia Vulgaris saps iron(on purpose) but be careful, so does walking...You can weaken your heart by taking too much Mugwort combined with walking...So use that Manganese herb judiciously...

Walk means walk...
About 2 hours worth of walking...If you are just starting to walk & you are very slow because you are out of shape or overweight because your hormones are wacky, then

make your walk 3 hours, but stop to pat dogs, chat or just look at the trees...(feel free to bring business cards if you are a networking addict-trail walking is a great networking place)...Goal is about 10 kilometres, 6 miles total...Yup it's far...No need for speed, take as long as you need...In fact walking fast is a drag...You'll get faster organically just because you become impatient...But slow is better really...Fewer injuries & more joy & more chances to chat with new people or dogs or birds or squirrels...Socializing while walking is fun...But walking alone is good...Walking in pairs or groups causes stress due to speed differentials...Try to walk alone...Meet other walkers, but be independent...Your speed choice is yours alone...Walking with others means you miss out on Nature & new experience...try to be brave...You are a RepoWoman after all aren't you?

Reward...

After your walk schedule a reward...This can change depending on the day, or can be the exact same thing...Sometimes I have a giant medium cappuccino with a free newspaper in a local cafe that is not a Starbucks at all but a place where non-chic people go...Sometimes I have a sashimi appetizer with a sunomo salad(crab, octopus, shrimp, seaweed, soya sauce, sesame seeds)...Yes, I cheat on my raw vegetable diet with fish & seafood...Cheating on your diet is good for the soul...If you allow yourself to cheat you will delight in the sneakiness of it all...Your cheating foods will taste even more delicious...You will feel like a rogue...RepoWomen know the rules & when to break them...Sometimes I buy myself something I don't need but like...Retail therapy is useful but if you are doing it all the time you may be going bipolar...Cut back on the Vitamin D3 if you are spending too much money...It's a trigger...One day I spend $25 at a tanning salon for a tan & the lotion stuff in a little cup...Felt like a million bucks after...Excellent reward, the warm rays make you feel great & your butt looks smaller the next day!(Don't do this often or your face will get wrinkly)...

Grocery Shop...
After your walk & reward you will be pretty tired...If you brought one of those fold into a tiny tiny ball type nylon-ish reusable bags, then you could have stuck this in your Fanny Pack before the walk...This means you can go from reward restaurant to grocery shop...If you didn't bring your bag, then go home, get your grocery bag(the reusable kind) & go back out to get your

groceries...Grocery shopping includes picking up any herbs you need, any supplements, drink, & all your raw vegetable salad ingredients...Pick up a protein too in case you will too dizzy & need to cheat with some more protein...our diet is IMPORTANT to your RepoWoman protocol...Like maybe most important thing...So grocery shopping is a big important job & you need to take TIME to do it well & do not rush that...Your food needs to be delicious & healthy & so on...You have to read labels & know when they are lying...Gluten free products taste yuck, just avoid glutens altogether if you can...Cheat if you must but just cheat with organic grain glutens...They taste better & are cheaper than the gluten free gluck...

DIY Chemo Notes:Read Book 6
 RepoWoman for the BASIC DIY chemo protocol...
But know this...

An UPPER like Licorice Root combined with a DOWNER like Madagascar Periwinkle, can cause an up & down effect in your body...

If you are smart & you are, then stagger these DIY chemo herbs so that you are taking the upper in the morning, & the downer in the evening...

The one in the middle, the Mugwort, you could take in the middle of the day maybe...

This is a much more esoteric way to take your chemicals(herbs), so if you do figure that all out, be PROUD of yourself for that...It ain't rocket science but it is still good that you get it...

Know the side effects of each herb & stop taking one or the other or the other if you are having problematic side effects that are not expected...

Expected side effects are the ones that are supposed to happen...

Iodine DOES make you feel tired...Know that...Iodine does make your period come early...Use a online period tracker if you still get your period to make yourself aware...Try not to take too much Iodine that could throw you into early menopause...That would suck...Similarly, exercising too much can induce early menopause & injury...Know that...

Ok end of the RepoWoman advice...ish...for now...

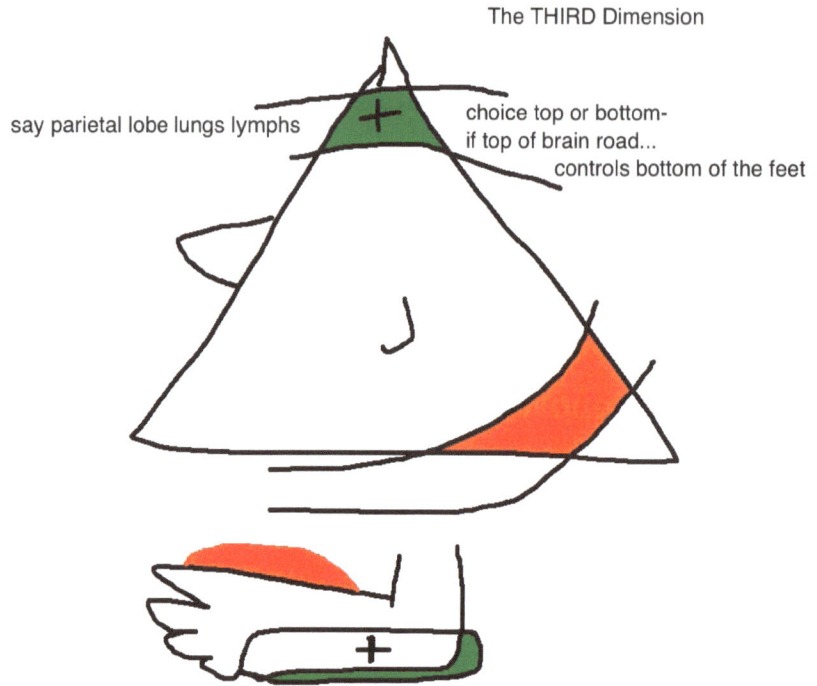

The THIRD Dimension

say parietal lobe lungs lymphs

choice top or bottom-
if top of brain road...
controls bottom of the feet

Third Dimension...Of paired brain parts...(where are they & which one is which)???

Choices are: one, two,& three...ASSUMING we are looking at a PAIR of brain parts...For the sake of argument there are 22 brain parts which makes 11 pairs, each pair controls one organ also known as a body part, in the case of paired body parts we might suppose that the BRAIN PART is One large piece like the Parietal lobe which one

SIDE of represents one FEATURE of the pair...In the case of brain parts that are separate but are INDEED paired, we might assume that each one of those separate brain parts like the globus pallidus & the hypothalamus CONTROL ONE body part (organ) that is SEEN as a whole like the SPLEEN...However with further study we might be able to say that the RIGHT side of the SPLEEN is MORE the Plus element side, & the left side of the spleen, the body part, the organ, is the Minus element side... So if we drink a cup of tea(Copper), we might think that the tea arrives mostly in the Left side of the Spleen, but maybe at the same time as it goes into your mouth it arrives at the Globus Pallidus too, since the Globus Pallidus sits IN FRONT of the Hypothalamus, WITHIN the PAIR...(relative to each other)...Everything is relative within pairs when looking for polarity(Minus or PLus element)...

Front of brain or back of brain...

Answer:Front brain Minus element, Back brain Plus element...

Left side of brain or right side of brain...

Answer:left side of brain Plus element...Right side of brain Minus element...

Top of brain or bottom of brain...

Answer(HOW we reasoned this out):If men like the bottom of their feet, then one might assume the top of the brain is a male dominant PLUS element area...If women like the TOP of their feet, how they look, how pretty their toenails are, THEN we might assume that the TOP of the feet are Female dominant...That means the BOTTOM of the brain is a MINUS dominant minus element place...

(Because the brain criss-crosses to the body part because the criss-cross is stronger...

We can see the Criss-Cross in the way the FLOW of a natural thing like a cup of tea with a spot of milk in it goes...Flows... Remember Page 86?

The reason the pyramid is so attractive to us, is because it is based on 3...

Question 1:Top of the brain or bottom of the brain...

Question Number 2:Left side of the brain or right side of the brain...

Question #3:Front of the brain or Back of the brain...

3 choices...

3 choices of polarity...

Within those 3 choices of polarity there are TWO (2) brain parts, or sides of one big looking brain part...

We are going to say there are 22 brain parts, or sides of one big brain part, that represent 11 body parts, because those 22 brain parts or sides are PAIRED...

Within EACH paired brain part, once you decide polarity(based on the 3 questions)...

Then TELL ME which PART of that PAIR is the MINUS element controller & which one is the PLUS element controller...

If I tell you Broca's Area & Wernicke's area are a PAIR of brain parts, & that Broca's area sits more to the FRONT of the Brain than Wernicke's which sits more to the back, & they are a pair that BOTH control the GALLBLADDER, THEN...

Then...
We can say that Broca's area is a Minus element controller unit...
Wernicke's area is a PLUS element controller unit...

If the Gallbladder contains the Minus element Magnesium & the Plus element Mercury, then we know that Broca's area controls Magnesium in the Gallbladder, & probably that Magnesium element is found in the BACK area of the body part called the Gallbladder...(because the back of the human body is more MINUS element dominant...Women like to look at their derrieres alot!)(back massage anyone? All the women say yes...)(Men are front of body oriented...Men are right side of body right hand oriented...Men are bottom of the

foot oriented...The foot fetish is a male habit...Bottom of the foot, the line of a heeled shoe...That whole thing, they like..."How beautiful are the feet of those...*"(this is actually referring to the bottom of the foot, the arch shape-even the **army does not like a 'flat-foot'-common knowledge!)
* is written by somebody in the Holy Bible, New Testament area who writes in a Male voice...

Families of elements that are similar but stronger or weaker than...
Lithium stronger than, Lead...

Boron, stronger than Copper...

Chlorine, stronger than Fluorine...

Oxygen, weaker than Helium...

Helium is stronger than Oxygen as a Minus element, which means it is at the Bottom of the Grove Body Part Chart...
But curiously, Helium is LIGHTER than Oxygen...Yes, something in the Minus elements is STRONGER if it is LIGHTER...Helium weighs less than Oxygen but is a stronger Minus element...A bigger Minus if you can get your head around that...So Helium SUBTRACTS MORE than Oxygen does...
If you serve a glass of Hydrogen & want it to be lighter in weight, you could add some Oxygen to it, bubbles...If you want it to be much much lighter, then you could add Helium to it...Hydrogen PerOxide is lighter than just plain water H2O...Hydrogen one molecule, Oxygen two molecules...Hydrogen per oxide means that for EVERY hydrogen molecule you have one oxygen molecule...Normal water you get TWO Hydrogen for every one

Oxygen...So by adding an extra Oxygen for every or PER Hydrogen molecule, you get More total Oxygen, so your glass is lighter as Hydrogen PerOxide...

If you imagine an imaginary glass of Hydrogen PerHelium, then that should be even lighter than the HydrogenPerOxide... Neat eh?

If you inhale Helium instead of Oxygen that is MORE of a MINUS than Oxygen...If Oxygen is a Minus element, like Fire is a Minus element, then Helium is even lighter, even HOTTER than Oxygen...

So now we know that stronger MINUS elements are HOTTER...

We should also assume that stronger Plus elements are COLDER...So Lithium should be COLDER than Lead(Plomb Pb)...

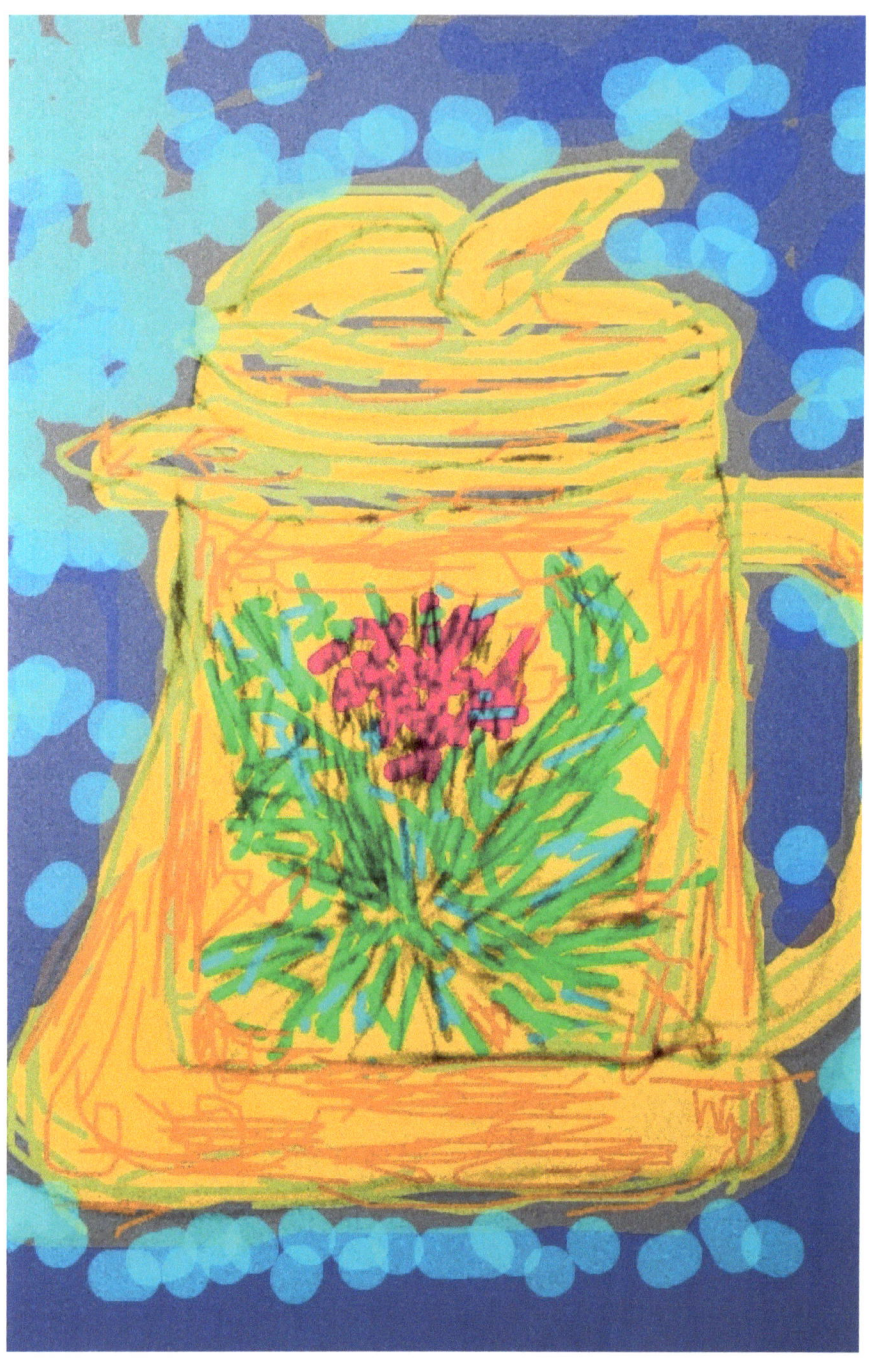

Chrysanthemum tea...

Zig Zag:

(do not go gently into that good night,)Rage
rage rage against the dying of the light,
Dylan Thomas...

I am ant vs; i am ant (notice the "i" is not
capitalized)...i forget

T.S.Eliot (what the Thunder said)

anon...

**Index credits...What follows is a flow (Feng Shui) of
thoughts that are variably UNedited...This is HOW I
come about getting new ideas & A-Ha moments...It is
an artist's technique sometimes called Abstract
Expressionism, (Les Automatistes) Automatism...**

ibid.

Zig Zag
Zig Zag Zig Zap poetry

Haiku

Letters...

Zig Zag means...(as a for example)

Magnesium Mercury
Fluorine Bismuth

Minus Plus
Minus Plus

(ok we are in the Gallbladder, then we are in the Colon)...

SINCE Minus comes first in the Order of Things...

Then Plus...

The female comes before the male, historically, in Evolution, in Creation, in Dinosaurs, first the female came first then the brave one dinosaur allowed his ovaries to drop out & be exposed, & hence the genitalia fell out & was not embarrassed...

Not embar-arr-assed to be seen...

To boldy boldly go where no man has gone before...(Star Trek William Shatner's speech aopning intro protion)(opening intro portion)...

Sorry dyslexia due to mercury excess in Gallbladder this morning due to poop in Balsmaic Vinaigrette o Lake Ontario soup...

Did you know the swirl of Lake Ontario swirls from a higher Great Lake to a Lower great Lake?

.> no more links<

However, in times of need, the Lake will swirl up the other way due to trouble below, south of us the States you idiot...(sorry, telepathy s a feature of the Holy Ghost, Mother Nature...)

An Inceberg could be made of Fluroine, Fluorine, Fluoride...Iceberg...F

Plus cement, Al;Aluminum.

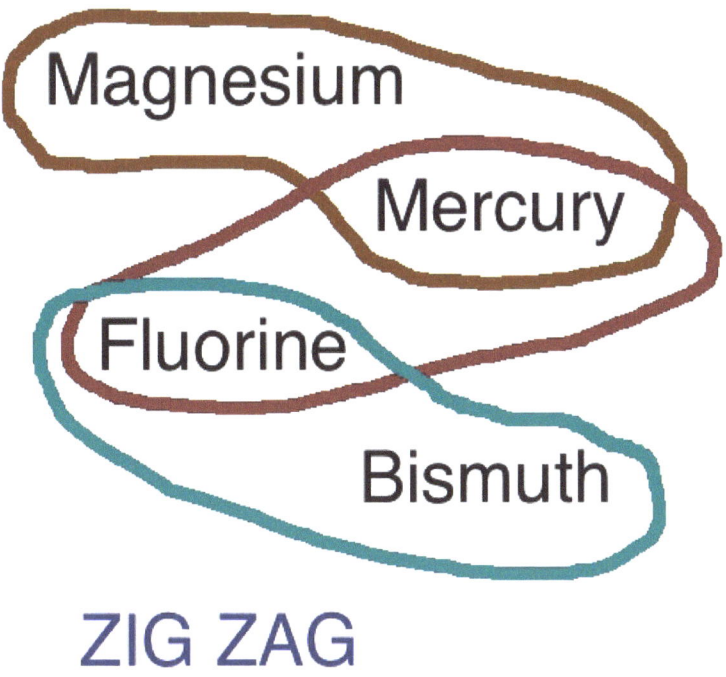

ZIG ZAG

Zig Zag means what the shape the SHAPE of the Body Parts the BODY PARTS are ARE...

(is there are echo in here, echolalia, echo-alia, echo, eco, umberto ecco)...

When you hit a mountain with your mouth (your words) it hits and creates an ECHO echo...

The body parts Zig Zag from Minus to Plus to Minus to Plus to Minus to Plus, NOT ad absurdium & NOT everything reduces down to carbon...

However it is useful in discusiion to end enerything with carbon because, discusiion typo, typographical, error, evrything, everything...

Stop...the telegrm stop...telegram stop...

The fStop Fstop on the camera...The stop...

Period. Ellipsis.Etc Etc...(and so on)

& I told two friends, egoiste(s) commercial.

Creve...CrevĖe9flqt tire in french gq,e; crevee accent aigu means flat tire or tired or je suis crevee, as in a metaphor...Too much carbon...Flat tire?

Tire is filled with Oxygen...O
Tire is filled with Nitrogen...N
Tire is filled with Helium...He
Tire is filled with crbon, Carbon C...

Tire is filled with he Helium lighter than Oxygen...But more likely to explode due to extreme lightness of Helium, variability with Oxygen, variability with Hydrogen in air...

Creates a 3 layer effect...Helium, Oxygen, Hydrogen...

Layered things are harder to kill but alos harder to biodegrade theoretically(in my opinion)...

Also...

When Helium comes in contact with Oxygen...

Oxygen feels upset because Helium weighs less & is so much skinnier & somebody has a pillow that says you can never be too rich or too thin but that is not true at all you can you can...

Too rich is greed, & too thin is anorexia or you are starving to death or you are so poor you cannot eat or afford food & you die & death is a sin so Ha!

Lazarus come forth...

Zig Zag...

Variability of weights of things(density actually)

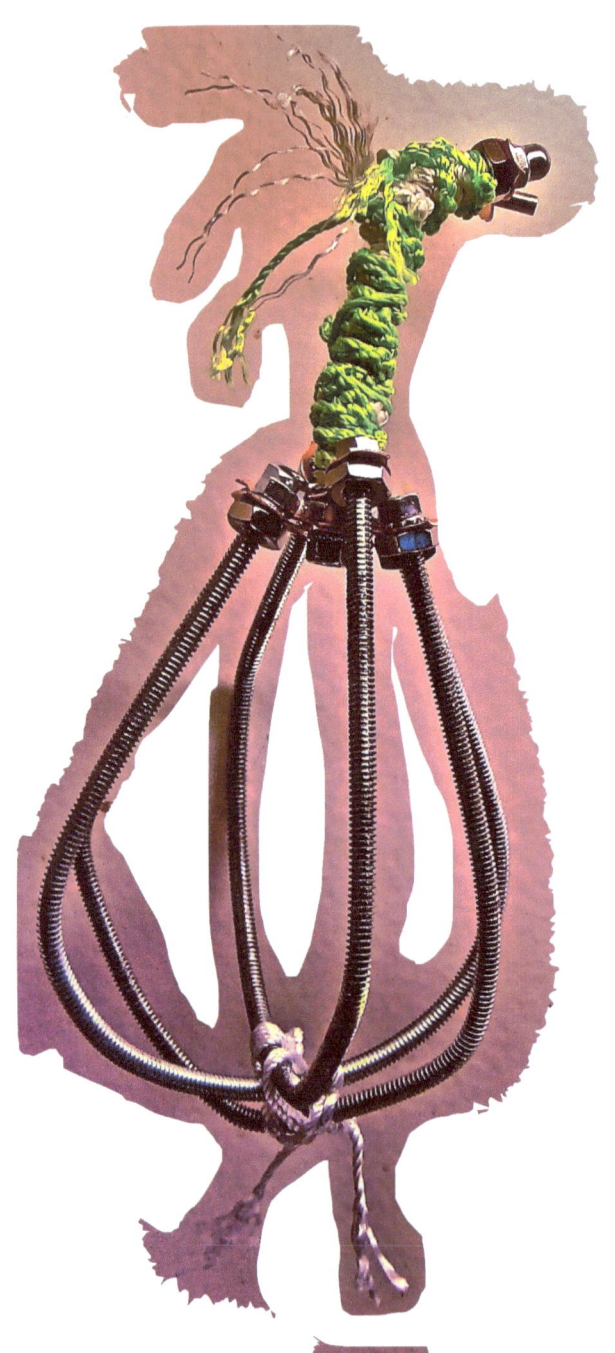

Grape on a Vine

(it looks like a Chardonnay, mustard coloured)

Facial scarring, cold weather, malaria, mosquito, left side of face, cutting, carotid artery, surgeon habit, picking of pimples or leaving them alone-Christian Science=leaving them alone because you picked them already & it is an annoying habit...

Habit, nuns...(free association)

"I was a nun until I kicked the habit!"(bada bump)(bum)...joke

Menmomics, songs, song lyrics, rhtym & rhyme. rhythm. rime of the ancient mariner-sad stopry spoler alert)(spoiler alert).

Mnemonic

G'd Night...(In the Night Kitchen by ...?)

Shel Silverstein Hug Me...)Porcupine in the forest at GPS left of the city Toronto & North of the City Toronto...On the trial trail thru the ...

Horses...Hoorsee...Mares? Cows. Cow car caa ...get your oil changed or I...threats...mechanic...(stanic mechanic) Stanislawvski cabbage.

Mihaly Chicksent mi haighy...feng shui flow football cte concussive traumatic encepahpolohpay elephant lephant man woman.

Hippopotamus left ankle basketball injury...

Tendon=Cartilage =Gallbladder=Mercury excess? I work out" " epub no spaces in image name.

Manesium is exercise...Magnesium...

Nitrogen reishi mushrooms? King/

The mushrooms in Connecticut have more Nitrogen in them than the mushrooms in Toronto because warning FALSE assumption follows- censor

The mushrooms in the park here are SUPPOSED to have more Nitrogen in them than the mushrooms in Connecticut(Yale) but they do NOT because the Yale ies stole our Nitrogen-it is called tha "brain drain here"...The the.

Tall new buildings is the name of a band.

Some of Sari Grove's raw in process artworks pictures(the underneath that is no longer visible once the works are finished)...See more at http:// www.grovecanada.ca

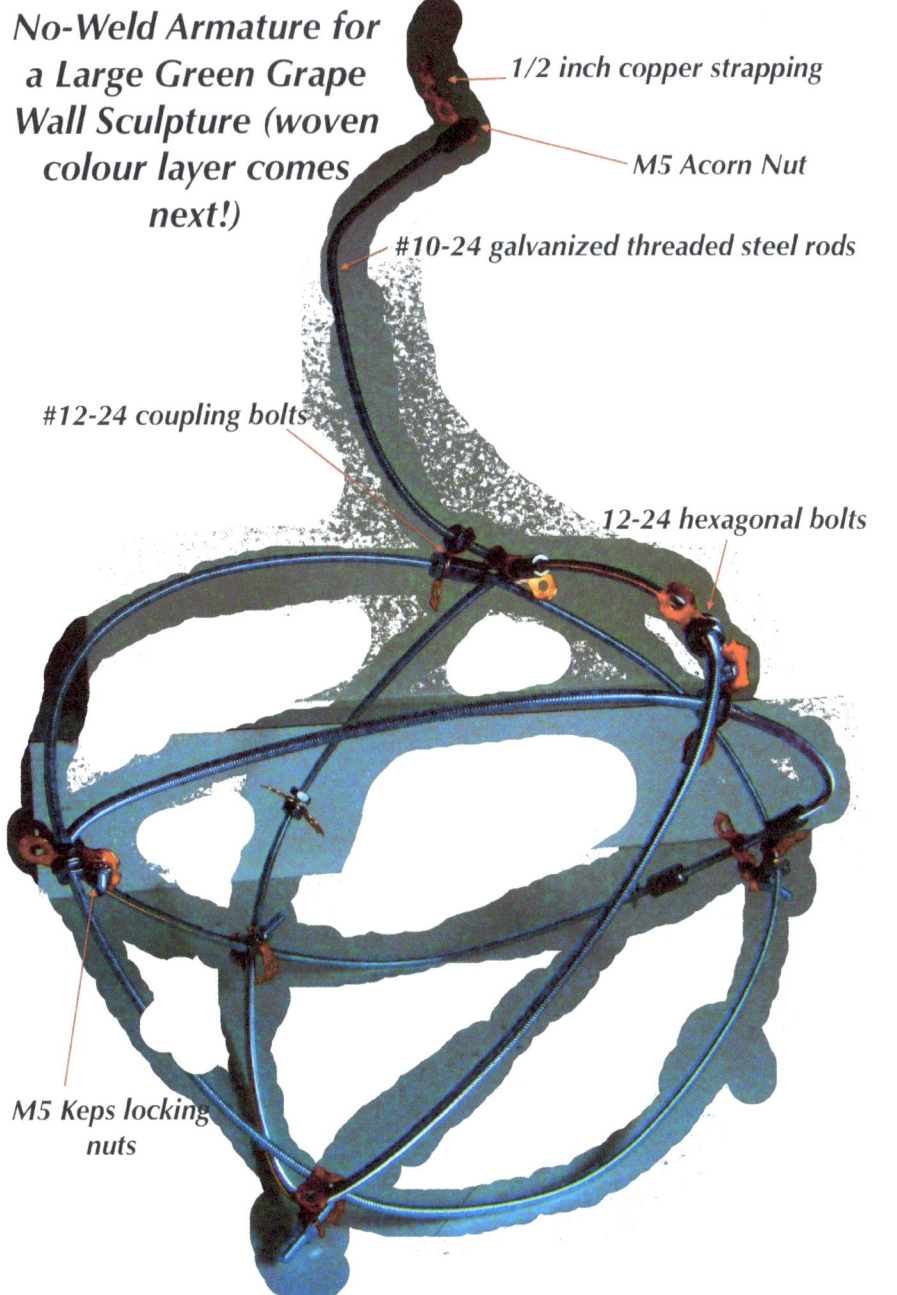

No-Weld Armature for a Large Green Grape Wall Sculpture (woven colour layer comes next!)

1/2 inch copper strapping

M5 Acorn Nut

#10-24 galvanized threaded steel rods

#12-24 coupling bolts

12-24 hexagonal bolts

M5 Keps locking nuts

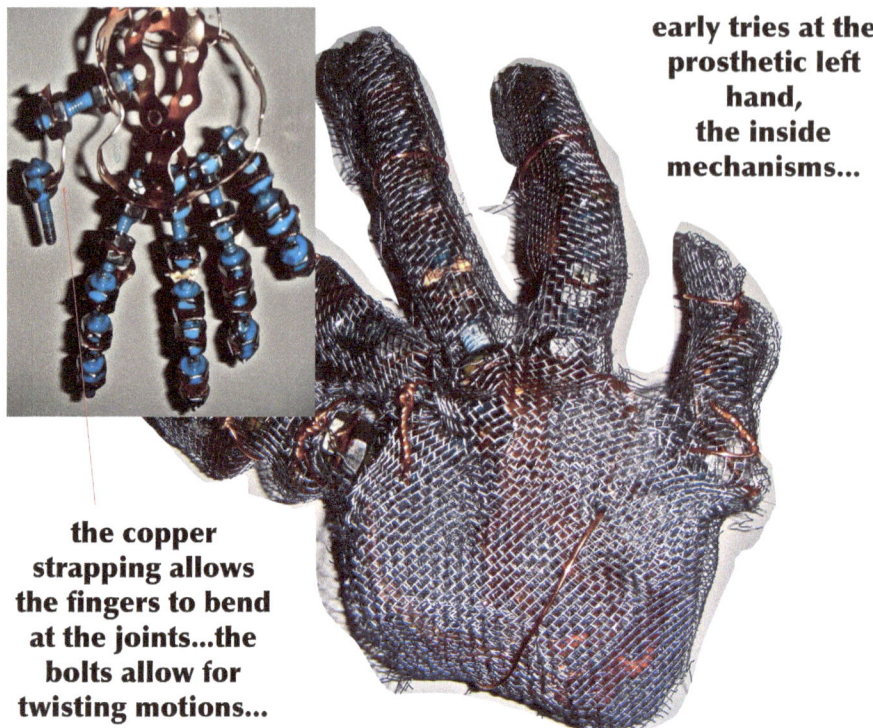

early tries at the prosthetic left hand, the inside mechanisms...

the copper strapping allows the fingers to bend at the joints...the bolts allow for twisting motions...

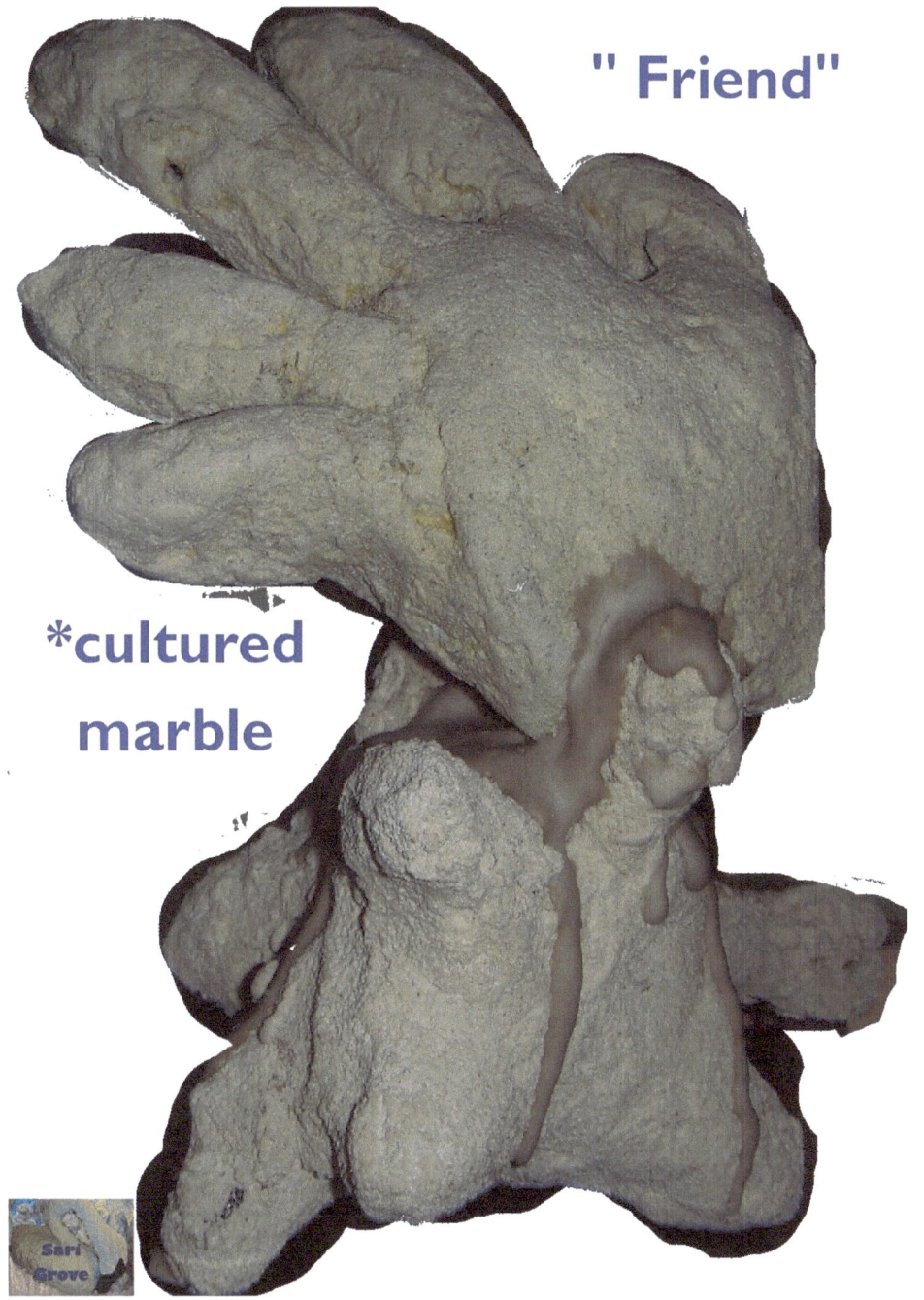

" Friend"

*cultured

marble

A second look at gender Polarity in brain & body parts...

Gender POlarity

direction BraintoBodyPart

**the left side of the brain part
controls the right body part
the top of the brain part in a pair
controls the Bottom of the feet for example
the front brain part in a pair
controls the minus element ie the female back of the body**

000

000

1111

1111

Fill in the Blanks...

Fill in the Blanks...

Frontal lobe r l means...
that the frontal lobe has 2 sides a right side &
a left side

Broca's area & Wernicke's area are paired...

are paired... Broca's sits to the front & Wernicke's area sits to the back (of the brain)

Broca's controls Magnesium production...

In the Gallbladder...

& Wernicke's controls Mercury production in the Gallbladder...

The Gallbladder makes Tendons Cartilage but NOT marbleing, not Aluminum, Not cholesterol, Not Fat...

A terrible terrible mistake...

Sarcasm... 01 0+1 0

0-1 0-1 , (0-1) turn tight turn right again go straight go left go left again go left again(you are now into a

go left again go left again(you are now into a SPIN) Fibonacci Alan Turing...credits.

Alan Turing pioneered the code for turning...When telling someone to turn right he would code that plus 1 or +1...Turn left was coded Minus One -1...Go straight was coded Zero 0...So when telling someone directions to his house he might say: "0, 0, 0, 0, +1, 0, 0, -1..."
Which would mean:"Go straight, go straight (each block), go straight, go straight, then turn right one block, then go straight one block, go straight another block, then turn left..."
There was an episode of the tv show Numbers that mentions this code...I learned it somewhere in high school (U.T.S.-The

University of Toronto Schools, class of 1984)...Probably in Physics...Anyways, I loved this code idea so much that it became a part of our Grove Body Part Chart...Minus & Plus...I could have used Female & Male...Yin & Yang...But I liked Minus & Plus because it has the least political incorrectness...Sure women might mind that I gave them the Minus designation, but it was easier for me to explain than the Male & Female components that you get at hardware stores, ie: the male plug is an 'outy' versus the female plug which is an 'inny'...

other things that need more pondering...

effects of each element on the body & brain...

http://wddty.com What doctor's don't tell you is a great source for people who want to know more about something sort of medical but need it in plain English...

hulled hemp seeds to cats...deworm...I found a teaspoon of hulled hemp seeds was very useful in deworming myself, **(Worms, like the Salmonella Typhi worm, can hole up in your breast lung tissue & cause Cancers-which is what makes cancer extra-tricky to solve-you have to deworm yourself-Hulled hemp seeds, like a teaspoon, are powerful dewormers-just remember they also cause memory loss, so be careful & use JUDICIOUSLY)...** Hemp is a Titanium like clove powder, the traditional dewormer...I wonder if my cats would eat hulled hemp seeds...Probably...I bet it would deworm them too, but I am not going to try it unless I am really stuck...But it is an idea...(I am not crazy about chemical cat dewormers)...

I am a member of ArtConcrete group through Yahoo Groups...Here is an excerpt of a conversation about using Aragonite sand from pet stores for your marble dust in concrete recipes...(or just homemade marble recipes...See our website http://www.grovecanada.ca for some of those recipes we invented ourselves!)

"Interesting!

The Aragonite Sand at Pet stores is also sometimes labelled Calcium Carbonate Sand too!

It is nice to work with because it is not dusty...

Kama Pigments the link you provided is a most excellent company & the owner answers emails directly & will handle special orders easily & with little grief...

Their products are great & he makes as much as he can himself, plus he is also an artist, so he speaks our language...(Though his Native language is french actually)...

His name is Vincent Deshaies...

(They are based in Montreal, province of Quebec, Canada...

Kama Pigments sells through AboveGroundArtsSupplies.com in Toronto, the store beside the Ontario College of Art & Design University OCADU)...

But he will sell directly to artists as well, or from their website...(in French or English)...

The thing about the Aragonite sand or calcium carbonate sand from pet stores is it is a Natural colour not pure white...

I am guessing Kama Pigments Calcium Carbonate is white white...

Kama Pigments also has metallic powders that can be mixed with Damar varnish as a surface look..."

Here is an email letter I wrote a while back while I was working on Book 3 of this series(Grove Health Science Series)...

"http://youtu.be/2IULrs6J9jU This is the video that explains the chart...

You will notice on the chart that each organ has both a Minus or Plus element...

Minus elements tend to detoxify, to cleanse...

Plus elements tend to nutrify or feed the body...

So in ailments where there is too much of a Plus element, like Cancer is too much calcium, you need to add that Minus to your life...

So the Iodine things...

Now in a general way, adding the other Minus elements will help to detoxify the whole body...

Now the thing about a calcium excess, Cancer or even benign breast cysts or lumps, or lumps anywhere, is that the Calcium gets stuck where there may be a buildup of another element too...

So if the lump ends up in the breasts, which sit on top of the lung lymph node system, then there may also be a buildup of that Plus element there too...

In the Lungs & Lymph nodes the Plus element is Aluminum...Which is why many breast cancer people stop using Aluminum deodorants...

The Minus element in the lungs & lymphs is Titanium...Titanium is found in aspirin, marijuana, hemp seed oil, Frankincense, that kind of thing...

So many people with breast calcifications will say rub Frankincense oil on their armpits & nipples too, with the Iodine...

Now calcifications can occur in any part of the body...

So the Iodine corrects the adrenal gland imbalance, & then you add the Minus element to target where that lump is...

Whey protein falls into the magnesiums...Magnesium is the Minus element in the Gallbladder...So, of course, adding magnesium helps to detoxify the Gallbladder-which is a big issue today because Magnesium antidotes Mercury, which is a big problem today because mercury can come from poopy water, poopy air, living near sewage treatment plants...

Which is why whey protein also works for autism adhd spectrum children & adults because those are mercury gallbladder problems...

Fungus is in the Leads, which is in the Thyroid gland...Aspergillosis too...MS too...Also lupus...So fungus is offset by the Minus there which is Zinc...Zinc is in sunshine, Vitamin D, ginger, turmeric...Which cleans out Thyroid Cancers...(with the Iodine)

So any potion or regimen that wants to clean the body out should contain the full list of Minuses...

Of course you have to be careful...

Too much detoxifying can bring new problems...

But you're right...Sugar for example is in the Sulphur category...Clogs up the Pancreas...

Alcohol is in the Liver & is a Hydrogen...

What is sad today is that people don't have to take birth control drugs anymore to be affected...

if you live in new York city for example, the water supply has enough birth control drug in the runoff to cause cancers...

There are male fish exhibiting female characteristics to the point of bearing eggs, who have merely been exposed to birth control drugs in their water..."

https://vimeo.com/91528571 Here's the video on Vimeo...Might be easier to watch than the Youtube one...

From September 2009, an early version of the chart...

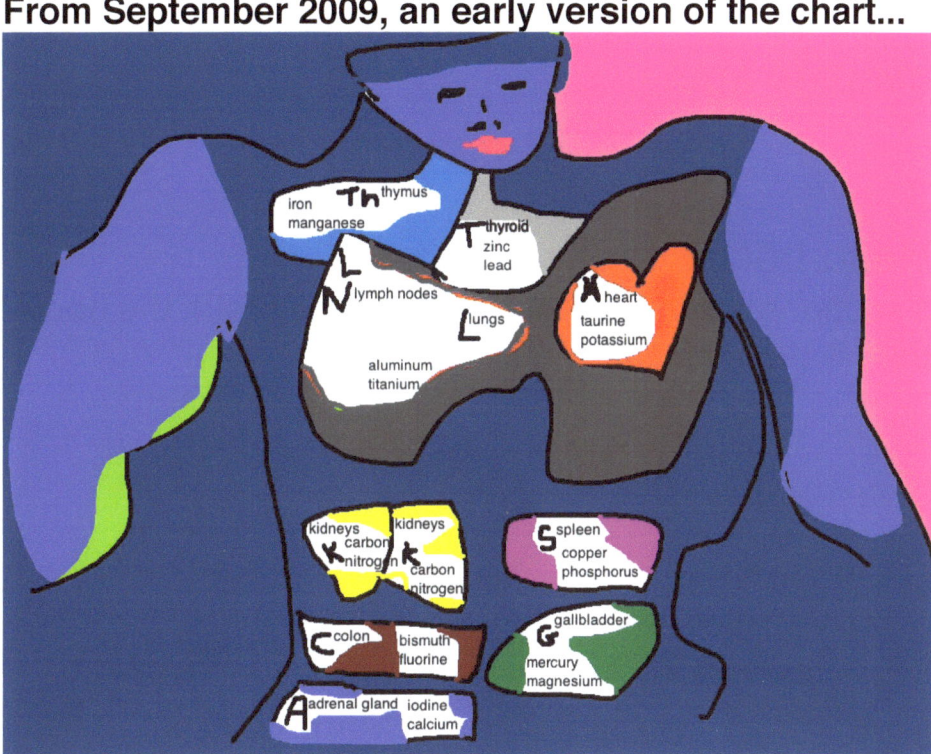

Food for thought...My rough notes to myself(I email ideas to myself,in the middle of the night, from bed, from my iPhone Notes app, to my Fastmail account, so I can see them in big on my desktop computer in the morning...)

Sari Grove <sari@fastmail.fm>

To:

grovecanada@fastmail.fm

Date:

Wed, 26 Nov 2014 6:02 AM (8 hours 33 minutes ago)

3
Head body limbs
3 sections(are there really 3 parts- the brain, the body part, & then the limbs???)

the 3 parts

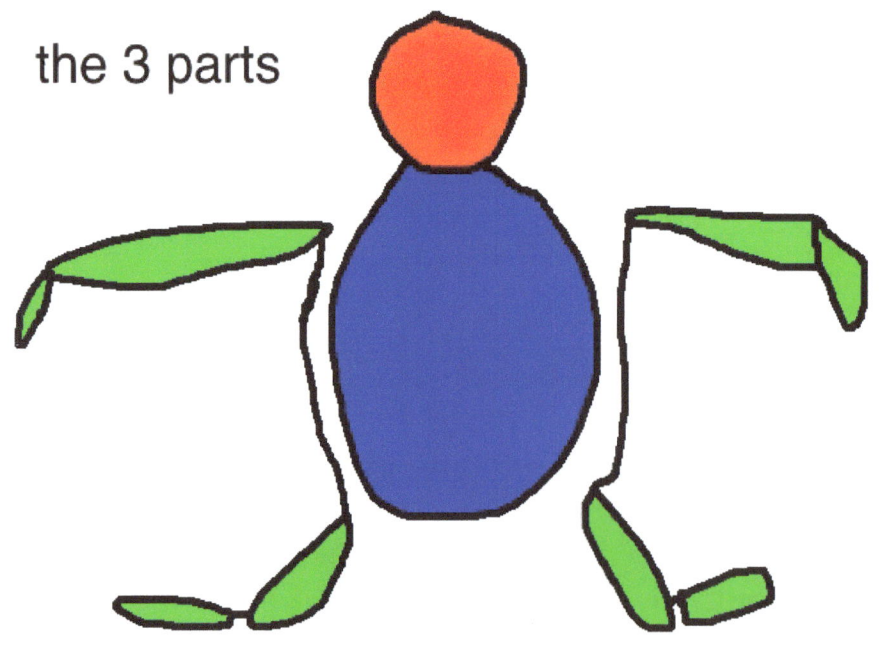

Ginger is lead antidotes lithium OZ
Suspect titanium memory loss affect

Premature ejaculator wet liver

Speak in c
Range high c
Low c range
Thoughts 2 floors up extra high c

Lack of sense of smell. Too much Oxygen
Febreze...

Hydration the spinal column the Liver

Down the lungs heart esophagus to
stomach thru colon intestines And so on
with bypass to gallbladder spleen etc then
out the anus with excrete or , out kidneys
pancreas back up spinal cord to brain at
back of Stem...

(that the body flow goes BACKWARDS or UP the spinal column to the Brain-that the body sorts through good & bad stuff when eating, excretes what it doesn't want, then what remains gets to go up the spinal cord, upwards to the brain stem, which is why only the most select items make it up to the brain-like Cilantro for instance Does make it up to the brain...)

In Front of Brain. Down (mouth), back upwards to stembrain! Brain stem in reverse.

Nicotine with burnt paper produces ash bismuth in lung forms extra skin (colon) plus element
(that the new e-cigarettes do NOT burn paper, so NO ash Bismuth goes into the Lungs...Is it the ASH in regular cigarettes that causes buildup of gunk?)

Oz contains Ti+Pb= memory loss cholesterol loss bone skeleton gain upper body breastplate (larger breast look ie)

(That ingesting Lead things like a potato or a carrot, builds that part of the body, like the Bones, & then that area will look bigger & be bigger...So like if you want to build your breastplate skeleton "look"...Eat things that are Plus elements in the Thyroid...)

Repeat what we know about Polarity...

Top of inside brain is bottom of the feet is male Plus element,

Bottom of inside brain part(of pair) is female,

So Pons is a vertical brain part at back of brain in brain stem,

Top of Pons controls then a Male Plus element of Kidneys(we know that) ,

So top of Pons controls right Kidney Nitrogen Plus element,

Left kidney is Carbon minus female element & bottom of Pons...

Because brain stem direction flows UP the back of the spine into brain, brain parts are backwards to body parts in polarity or direction...

Sulphur sugar is ideas China sugar excess diabetes blindness no peripheral vision William Gibson Peripheral (new book people are reading by the same person who invented the word cybernetics, & wrote The Matrix film scripts...)

Mastyrbating to release excess Phosphotus is like exercise
(idea:that releasing Phosphorus by masturbation lowers testosterone levels or estrogen levels, also thus lowering violent impulses, since violence has been linked to high testosterone levels...)

Sec x is fog dpkdport for sport(that sexual activity is a sport)

Go slow to go fast...
Slow down to go faster!(planning to drive slowly in heavy traffic or construction relieves the anger associated with that trip & makes the rest of the day seem to go faster & easier...Plus going slower in ALL things that you do enables fewer mistakes & edits later...Which is faster in the long run...)

Teaspoon hemp seeds important!
For bug removal

Bismuth Pepto Bismol antidotes fluorine date rape drug and hangover
(that the Bismuth in Pepto Bismol is great hangover remedy because much of the liquids we drink contain Fluorine which causes diarrhea & vomiting...Bismuth antidotes fluorine...)

Hydrogen is the mechanism that puts you to sleep alcohol blacking out

(that when you "black out" when drinking heavily, it is the Hydrogen just putting you to sleep...Which is why insomniacs like drinking...water, alcohol, whatever that contains Hydrogens...Oxygens wake you up...)

Blackened foods ash bismuth African cooking barbecue. Big giant teeth no fluorine problems Sari

(that people of African origin have great teeth due to high Ash Bismuth consumption because they eat foods more likely to be blackened over a flame...Consider eating more barbecued foods if your teeth are thin over-fluoridated looking?)

Sent from my iPhone

p.s.This book(& all the others too) gets edited & updated from time to time...Raw versions as we progress are available all the way along because that is the world we live in today...Immediacy is the norm & people don't want to wait 10 years anymore for medical information to be released...

Problems...

Water flowing backwards...

On Sundays, it seems that the dentist's offices clean out their old fluoride syrups...At the same time, on Sundays, people seem to use less water...Then there is some sort of a backdraft happening, where when you run your water taps, the dredge from the dental office comes out your outflow water taps...Weird eh? & sort of gross! I noticed it in our condo, & also when I had a CocoMint creme tea at David's tea at Yonge & St. Clair...Had a fluorine effect after I drank it...

Wonder when dentist's will stop overfluoridating our Lake Ontario water supply???

Febreze contains Oxygen...Spray on cat pee spots & the smell just disappears! neat!

Cayenne Pepper, a Selenium element, reverts to a lesser Minus element when cooked-ie Turmeric, a Zinc on our chart...So

when you cook something it has less power...
Radon(think radiation) is a Zinc element , just stronger on the Periodic Table of Elements...

Take a picture of all your computer connections, DVD burner, TV set connections, PVR, Airport...Later, when you upgrade you might actually be able to reconnect things!

End of Lucky Book 7:Homework Textbook for the Keen Medical Mind, for now...

(Wed. Nov. 26, 2014)

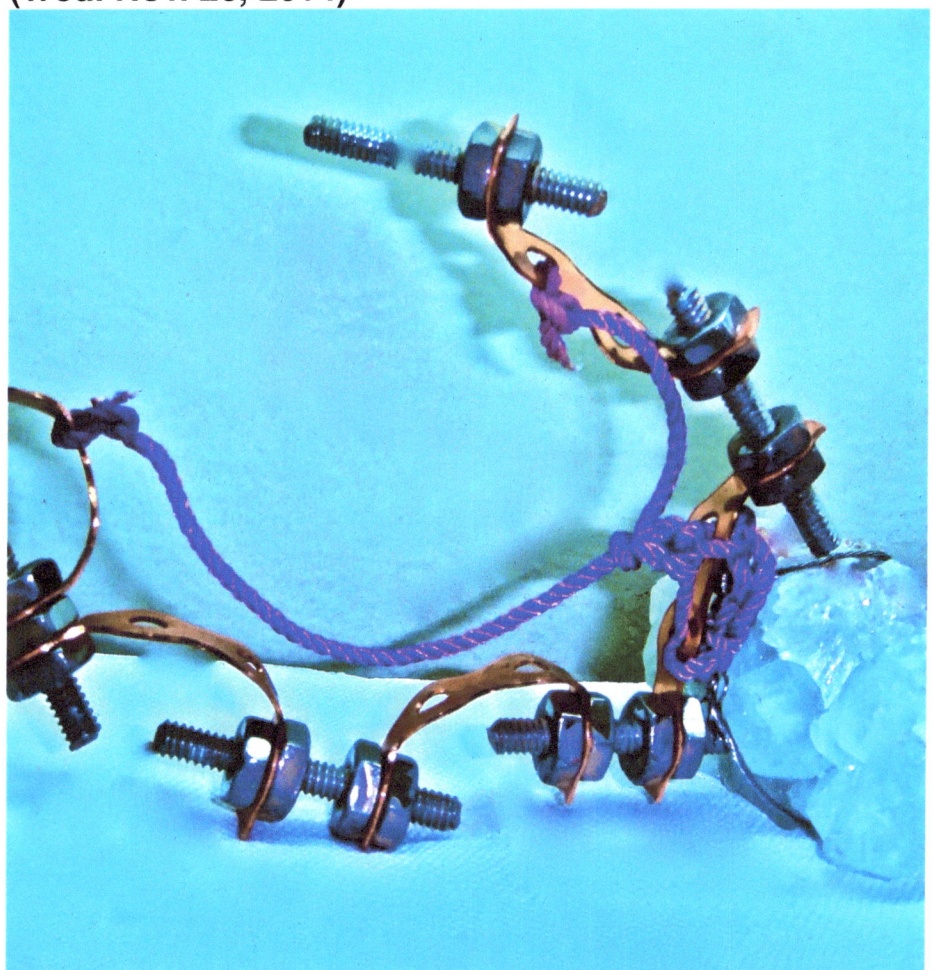

The Making of a prosthetic left hand...Sari Grove

www.ingramcontent.com/pod-product-compliance
Lightning Source LLC
Chambersburg PA
CBHW040755200526
45159CB00026B/2607